Herbalism

How to Improve Your Health by Using Inexpensive Accessible Herbs

(Create Your Herbalist Apothecary With Accessible Natural Herbal Remedies)

Samuel Unger

Published By **Oliver Leish**

Samuel Unger

Herbalism: How to Improve Your Health by Using Inexpensive Accessible Herbs (Create Your Herbalist Apothecary With Accessible Natural Herbal Remedies)

ISBN 978-1-998927-59-3

No part of this guidebook shall be reproduced in any form without permission in writing from the publisher except in the case of brief quotations embodied in critical articles or reviews.

Legal & Disclaimer

Table Of Contents

Chapter 1: The History of Herbalism

When confronted with illnesses and health troubles, the human race has needed to come up with approaches of retaining themselves healthful and thriving. From the beginning of time, viruses, infections, accidents, and ailments have been and however are the largest enemy of mankind.

In the look for solutions, our ancestors have encounter flowers. They started out out searching their animals devour them and perplexed whether or not or no longer or not it turn out to be sincerely well really worth investigating and the use of them to heal their sick ones.

In this bankruptcy, we can be looking at Herbal medication at some stage in information, from the primary historic records of humanity's findings to the cutting-edge-day herbalists who benefit from said findings and preserve to characteristic new records to the list thru the technological information we call

Botany. To create an knowledgeable and sensible view on what herbalism is and its blessings, we want to be aware about the beyond and what it teaches us about the way people noticed it for loads of years and the way their view changed thru the centuries.

Herbalism has its roots deep in antiquity, predating written human data. And as we can not be tremendous of methods all of it began out we will anticipate that women were the ones to first exercising it.

In the early historical times, guys were the hunters and women the gatherers. They should use everything they may discover in nature to cook dinner, make clothing, and heal ailments. We can count on that to parent out what is toxic and what's secure they had to have a look at animals and talk with distinctive ladies about their findings. If a person may also are becoming poisoned, they may understand which plant to keep away from. As that is best hypothesis because of the fact there is no written proof of this being actual, many scientists take shipping of as genuine with it to be very probable giving the way historical families needed to divide hard work.

The first written record of vegetation used for a medicinal purpose became created over 5 thousand years inside the past by using the Sumerians, on clay pills in present day Iraq or the ancient Mesopotamia. They created lists of loads of medicinal plant life collectively with opium and myrrh. The writings display us nowadays the importance of vegetation to our historic ancestors. They taken into consideration their discoveries without a doubt really worth writing down regardless of the reality that, writing in those times became scarce and difficult. It indicates us the form of recognize the Sumerians had for plant life and their ability benefits.

A few millenniums later, for the duration of the only yr 1500BCE, the Ancient Egyptians wrote a report known as the "Papyrus Ebers" list over 850 herbal drugs we apprehend and use in recent times.

The Papyrus lists illnesses and treatments from "sickness of the limbs" to "ailment of the pores and skin". Some of the flowers listed as treatments had been garlic, juniper, cannabis, castor bean, aloe, and mandrake. In the way they have been writing, the signs regarded to be seemed as the infection itself and the treatments were aimed closer to treating the signs. Scientists do no longer doubt that the Papyrus file changed into carried throughout the location via exchange and politics, influencing and evolving the way many cultures perceived medication. Some tomb illustrations and jars containing traces of herbs additionally function proof for the ones findings.

Looking at historic Egyptians these days we can be extremely good they possessed terrific statistics in numerous subjects as they used to put in writing down on stone everything they deemed important and we will look at and translate nowadays the hieroglyphs to research from their cultures. The Papyrus writings regarded to be of wonderful importance to them, as they made nice to keep it very carefully. Most of their understanding of drugs and illnesses were being registered inside the ones historical books. The understand they had for vegetation is simple and their discoveries on their usefulness concerning signs seem to be simple.

In India, round 4000 BC Sanskrit writings collectively with the Rig Veda and Atharva Veda have been some of the earliest writings that formed the concept of the Ayurveda tool, one of the oldest restoration structures. It changed into primarily based on the notion that fitness and fitness rely upon the stability a number of the body, mind, and spirit. This gadget used turmeric collectively with many distinct herbs and minerals defined by using way of the use of historic Indian herbalists like Charaka and Sushruta at some point of the 365 days one thousand BC. Indians seemed to have been the primary ones who understood the importance of plants in recovery, to this point in order that they built an entire restoration tool round it.

In historical China, a mythological Chinese emperor named Shennong is stated to have written the primary Chinese pharmacopeia, the "Shennong Ben Cao Jing", list 365 medicinal plants and their uses, inclusive of Ephedra, a shrub used to introduce ephedrine to trendy remedy, hemp and chaulmoogra, one of the first powerful treatments for leprosy.

From historic times, the Chinese have saved their herbalist traditions, being the most vital herbalist network within the global in our modern-day-day times. They despite the fact that workout natural treatment and use remedies they have got identified to paintings for loads of years. They use herbalism along side Western medicine and they defend their our our bodies the usage of plant life earlier than they even get. So in location of going to the clinical medical doctors after illnesses have already got an impact on their our our bodies and fitness, they go to the doctors extra frequently and use plant-based totally remedies and treatments to strengthen their our bodies and defend them from feasible illnesses and diseases. We ought to be aware about japanese treatment and their practices due to the fact they must have stored their traditions for a motive.

One of the famous if no longer the most famous physicians of all time is Hippocrates. He lived amongst 460-377 BC in Greece and believed that our our our bodies have become diseased certainly and the illnesses have been now not because of superstitions or with the aid of manner of God, in comparison to the popular perception within the ones days. While in prison for containing opposing perspectives to the authorities of his days, he wrote the book "The Complicated Body" which consisted of many medical theories considered proper these days, and he's regularly known as the "Father of

Modern Medicine ". The Hippocratic Oath is being obsessed with the resource of the ones who whole medical degrees in our modern-day-day-day days. He used many herbal capsules and said the famous words"allow your meals be your drugs, and your tablets your meals". He wrote about the willow bark and its houses, giving the facts scientists needed to synthesize the active compounds of willow to make aspirin.

The Hippocratic Corpus grow to be composed of many writing and books which are related to Hippocrates and his findings, it modified into written with the resource of every Hippocrates and those who found and respected his manner of perceiving remedy. Though some of the plant life said in The Hippocratic Corpus have been similar to the ones utilized by religious sectors of restoration, they differ within the reasoning in the returned of the usage of them. That being logical and experimental, similar to Hippocrates used to suppose. He meant to offer plants the medical-based totally definitely sincerely recognition using his sensible and herbal way of seeing medicinal drug. Western treatment itself changed into based totally totally on plants and scientists these days are in the way of proving the high-quality consequences plant life have on the human body.

We will preserve to test ancient Greece and Rome and the folks who made excellent discoveries in natural medication.

Galen of Pergamon, a Greek physician working within the path of in Rome wrote many books at the medicinal use of plants with one of the most superb being "Works of Therapeutics". In this e book, he was discussing the connection among many disciplines and remedy and the way they are able to paintings together to restore people's health and properly-being. He moreover completed a very vital characteristic in Humoralism, a device of medicine created to detail the make-up and the workings of the human body. His role on this gadget changed into critical for a manner pharmacists placed out to arrange their treatments after statistics how every human frame is awesome.

Diocles of Carystus have become a Greek scientific medical health practitioner and author who lived near Hippocrates' instances. He grow to be referred to as the second one Hippocrates due to his complete paintings and similarity to Hippocrates' views. He is concept to have written the primary scientific e-book difficult the proof for this has been lost. However, his work changed into said in hundreds of cutting-edge scientists' writings further to his contemporaries' gaining sufficient understand to have his advice on herbal medication taken appreciably.

Pliny the Elder become a Roman author, naturalist, and natural truth seeker. He wrote the e-book "Natural History" as a complete manual to nature, offering an extensive catalog of herbs precious to medicine. This catalog with over 900 listed drugs and plants, brings high-quality fee to our modern-day-day know-how of herbal remedy, popularity at the base of what we understand approximately nature and its recuperation competencies.

Pedanius Dioscorides, stepping on Pliny's steps, a first-rate medical doctor himself, wrote some different pharmacopeia referred to as "De Materia Medica" because of this "Of clinical subjects". The books embody over 1000 drugs constituted of herbs, minerals, and animals. The treatments in the pharmacopeia had been widely used through historical times, making Dioscorides an expert on drugs for almost millenniums after his demise.

Theophrastus' e-book "Historia Plantarum" is also actually surely really worth bringing up inside the data of herbalism as it emerge as the first systematization of the botanical global. These Greek and Roman philosophers and scientists have been those who spread Herbalism and the data they collected finally of the whole international. We will study how their discoveries impacted remedy for the severa years to come beginning inside the Middle Ages.

Through the Middle Ages, the monasteries in Britain and mainland Europe commenced retaining herbalism. Monasteries have been serving as clinical schools earlier than the popularity quo of universities in the 11th and 12th centuries. Monks have been transcribing and copying the works of Galen, Dioscorides, and Hippocrates at the equal time as growing the maximum common and beneficial herbs of their "Physick" gardens to teach the following technology of clergymen and destiny physicians.

The nun monasteries had been furthermore looking for to spread the information of the historical physicians on plants as remedies for ailments. We can anticipate the motive monasteries took over as places of restoration for people might have been based absolutely totally on their non secular beliefs as flowers were applied in antiquities thru way of pagans and witches. There is evidence that the Christian Church has attempted through records to take over the practices of pagans and witches and offer them to God in a brand new and less superstitious way.

In the sixth and seventh centuries, after the Islamic conquest of North Africa, many eastern pupils have received the scientific writings of the Greeks and Romans. Avicenna, an Iranian medical doctor, combined the writings of Galen and Dioscorides on herbal treatment with those of his personal human beings and wrote "The Cannon of Medicine". The Cannon of Avicenna unfold through Europe within the eleventh and twelfth centuries and is considered one of the maximum influential texts ever written. The History of Medicine makes an crucial reference to Avicenna's work as the basis for treatment and herbalism mainly.

After the invention of the printing press in the mid fifteenth century, the natural remedies of Dioscorides, Galen and Avicenna began out to be carefully produced and bought outside the palaces, monasteries, and universities. The use of the natural capsules didn't require particular competencies, the readers should acquire the herbs and exercising them as prescribed.

In the ones instances there had been many writers who've been trying to find to revolutionize medicine and discover new plant-primarily based absolutely remedies. One of the most famous ones became Paracelsus (1493-1541). He emphasized the affected person experience and how ignorant it might were to conform with blindly the historical physicians.

Even no matter the truth that he made very easy his distrust in traditional herbalism, Paracelsus brought lower back to life the 1st-century "doctrine of signatures" which said that every plant has its specific sign. It explains how the colour, form, look, and environment of a plant suggests it is medicinal use. For instance, the pansies with their coronary coronary heart-commonplace petals have been used for coronary heart problems. This doctrine of signatures have become recognized with the aid of manner of the physicians of in recent times and commenced out gaining popularity in the western international.

Englishman, Nicholas Culpeper, a century later, revived a few exclusive historical a part of herbalism: astrology. In astrological herbalism, herbs have been connected to zodiac symptoms and signs and symptoms and signs. They treated illnesses thru looking on the a part of the body affected and finding the sign or planet that dominated over it. Then they could prescribe a herb that dominated under the equal astrological signal. Culpeper said that "He that could comprehend the purpose for the operation of the Herbs, ought to look up as high because of the truth the stars."

Medical exercise started out changing at the same time as Paracelsus and Culpeper were selling signatures and astrology together with herbalism. Men collectively with Francis Francis 1st Baron Beaverbrook and William Harvey have been changing era into an experimental machine, leaving inside the back of its speculative nature.

This end up the factor wherein organic and scientific generation commenced to separate from traditional herbalism. As the herbalists had been attempting to find to restore ancient practices, the medical scientists had been beginning to revolutionize the way technology modified into perceived completely. This distinction in motive is what split treatment into specific training.

From there, herbalists who refused to acknowledge the signatures and the celebrities however focused on class commenced the technological knowledge called Botany.

Physicians who taught Harvey's blood circulate idea became more useful than Cupeper's astrology idea, commenced what nowadays we name medical treatment.

The discoveries made inside the middle a while with the useful resource of technique of these super guys are taken into consideration milestones inside the records of Western natural medicine. From the principle deliver, the historical herbalists, to its glide from clinical era.

Looking at how medical remedy separated from traditional herbalism it's miles hard to accept as actual with clearly one in every of them is probably incorrect. Maybe it would have been higher for experimental remedy to mix with the conventional herbalism and shape a more complete way of searching at restoration. Something is sure, however, the fact that herbs play an essential position in healing and their importance desires to be said in every a part of the world.

Traditional herbalism has started to be seen as a way of possibility remedy in the United States and the Western worldwide in stylish for the reason that 1910 at the equal time because the Flexner Foundation released a report addressed to all clinical institutions, defining the manner medicinal drug need to be practiced and taught. The e book changed into known as the Flexner Report and it led all eclectic clinical faculties wherein botanical treatment emerge as absolutely practiced, to close for top.

In the Eastern global, Mao Zedong reintroduced into the health care system the Traditional Chinese Medicine that is based totally completely closely on herbalism, in 1949. Since then, the colleges have been schooling thousands of practitioners within the fundamentals of Chinese medicine, to workout it in hospitals. Hundreds of Americans fly to China to get an education in Chinese Medicine which suggests us that there are numerous health practicers unhappy with the authorities's desire over a century in the beyond.

In 1930 The UK end up experiencing issues inside the exercising of herbalism, stemming from the distinction from clinical medicinal drug. The United States began out out prohibiting the workout across the identical time. The World Health Organisations is estimating that approximately eighty% of people depend upon natural treatment for some a part of their health care. Germany has over 600 plant-based ones to be had and over 70% of physicians are prescribing them there.

Even even though throughout the vicinity the exercising of prescribing remedies and pills to staying power is relying on a medical license, no law prohibits the prescriptions or advice of plant-based totally totally treatments to anyone.

Looking at the sector nowadays, there is however a cut up among Western and Eastern remedy. In the Eastern worldwide, and additional specially China, traditional herbalism is being preserved and used each day by the usage of manner of the sufferers and prescribed with the aid of using way of the doctors. It is a massive part of their way of life and their national delight.

The Western worldwide is popping their lower again toward the workout and the scientists are focusing their efforts on experimental based absolutely remedy whilst forgetting frequently of the blessings plant life have at the human body.

It might be properly really worth searching at each manner of existence and locating the blessings from every of their scientific practices. One element is effective although, herbal medicine despite the fact that performs a totally crucial role in maximum of the arena's population and fitness.

Chapter 2: Popular Herbs Known to Improve Health

Herbs are embedded in the forefront of records. For masses of years, they had been fused into wealthy traditions and cultures anywhere in the global. The medicinal homes of these plant life are although very applicable these days. You may likely have come upon a number of those famous herbs even as on foot thru a lawn or have some growing to your outside. Here are some of those well-known herbs widely diagnosed for enhancing health.

1.Burdock

•Scientific call: Arctium lappa

•Origin: notwithstanding the reality that this plant is neighborhood to Asia and Europe, many species of burdock have been unfold anywhere within the international. Today, you could discover it growing in fields, empty regions, and roadsides all through North America, China, Britain, Europe, and different continents.

•Description: the burdock fruit is tough and ovate with prickly heads. The burrs annoyingly dangle to garb and fur. The burdock plant is broadly taken into consideration a weed inside the United States but it's far cultivated in Asia for the delicious root utilized in Korean and Chinese cuisine.

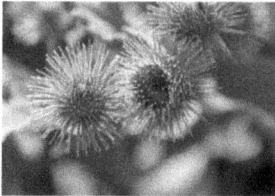

Some species of burdock can have their leaves increase up 28 inches extended.

2.Calendula

•Scientific call: calendula officinalis

•Origin: the lovely calendula flower is of northern Mediterranean origin. Its call is gotten from a Latin word 'kalendae' meaning the primary day of a month. This might be concerning the fact that calendulas bloom on the start of just about each month of the three hundred and sixty 5 days in community areas.

•Description: notwithstanding the truth that calendula flowers are commonly called pot marigold, this herb need to no longer be mistaken for vegetation in the marigold genus. Its super golden yellow and orange shade has been used for everything from

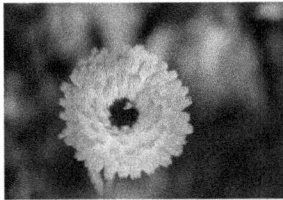

fabric coloring to meals and redecorating statues in Hindu temples.

3.Chickweed

•Scientific name: Stellaria media

•Origin: chickweed originates from Eurasia in Europe however has now been naturalized all around the international.

•Description: is a perennial and annual flowering herb from the circle of relatives

Caryophyllaceae. It is a low growing plant with small leaves on erect stalks that can amplify as lots as 18 inches tall. Chickweed yields white, small, famous person-fashioned

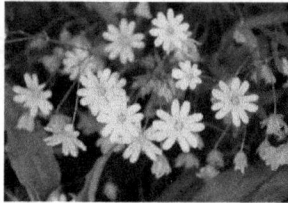

flora nearly all year round.

4.Dandelion

•Scientific call: Taraxacum officinale

•Origin: at the begin local to Eurasia, dandelions are virtually common in South America, North America, New Zealand, Australia, India, and lots of various areas that Europeans have migrated to. The English call is gotten from the French name 'dent de lion' because of this the lions teeth. This refers to the serrations like tooth on the plant's leaves.

•Description: Although many humans expect dandelion is only a weed, it is been cultivated for herbal remedies for a long time. The leaves expand from the crown of the plant, they're basal. The stalk can develop as much as 70cm tall and a milky latex oozes out if the

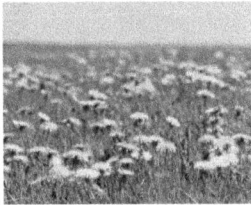

stem is damaged.

five.Echinacea

•Scientific call: Echinacea purpurea

•Origin: this flowering herb is indigenous to North America. Its earliest species can be traced lower again to Missouri and Arkansas from wherein it traveled in the route of the east in the Seventies. European researchers made echinacea well-known in 1939 while research had been completed on aerial factors of the plant.

•Description: additionally known as coneflowers, echinacea is a flowering herb from the daisy own family that has stunning purple petals. The petals surround a cone or

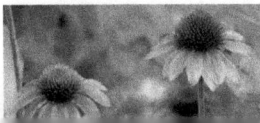

seed head product of darkish brown or reddish spikes.

6.Elderflower

•Scientific call: Sambucus nigra cerulea

•Origin: this hedgerow plant is nearby to areas of Europe and Britain. The elder tree, from which elderflowers broaden, is a quick-growing tree with flora present from June to July and leaves from March to November each 12 months. The facts of elderflower is going over again to the time of Greek doctor Hippocrates in four hundred BC.

•Description: the recognition of the elderflower plant has grown substantially within the past few years. Although there are rich history and hundreds of folklore approximately the herb, public interest in it peaked after it changed into added as one of the additives for Prince Harry and Megan Markle's royal wedding ceremony cake.

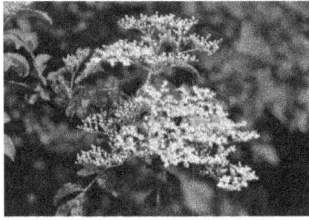

7.Nettle

•Scientific name: Urtica dioica

•Origin: this perennial flowering herb is neighborhood to Northern Africa, North America, Asia, and Europe. Nettle now grows all over the international mainly in North America and New Zealand.

•Description: do now not allow the beautiful coronary heart-fashioned leaves fool you, nettle, or stinging nettle, can provide you with a bristly rash on the identical time as your exposed pores and skin brushes upon it. Its leaves and stems are included with trichomes or stinging hairs that supply chemical acids to motive the stinging sensation. Thankfully, this endearing plant loses its sting whilst boiled to release nutritious tonic results.

eight.Oats

•Scientific call: Avena sativa

•Origin: probably originating from East Asia, oats date as an extended manner lower once more as 2000 BC after they were weeds. They had been first cultivated for medicinal abilities earlier than they had been grown for meals. Today, they are broadly farmed in lots of temperate regions.

•Description: bridging the divide amongst food and herbs, oats are a vintage restorative tonic. Oats, or wild oats, are from the grass own family and one of the healthiest grains inside the global. The annual plant can expand as a whole lot as five toes tall. This difficult plant can grow in sandy, alternatively acidic, low fertility soil provided there can be

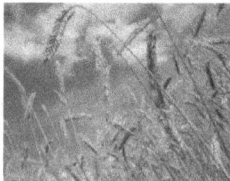

sufficient water.

nine.Peppermint

•Scientific call: Mentha x Piperita

•Origin: this hybrid herb is a bypass amongst spearmint and watermint plant life of the mint circle of relatives initially from Asia and Europe. Peppermint is now extensively grown in lots of additives of the arena and additionally may be decided developing in the wild.

•Description: peppermint is specifically valued for its flavor and it has many medicinal traits as well. It capabilities opposite growing leaves with jiggered edges and a crowning flower. Peppermint leaves can growth up to three.Five inches tall at the same time as the red flower only grows 0.31 inches tall. The flowering season for this aromatic herb lasts from mid-summer season to late summer season.

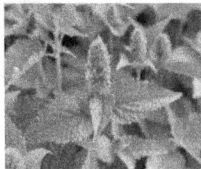

10.Yarrow

•Scientific call: Achillea millefolium

•Origin: this flowering plant of the aster circle of relatives originated from the temperate areas of Western Asia and Europe but is now popularly grown in New Zealand, Australia, and North America. The call achillea is referred to as after the Greek hero Achilles who used the herb to cope with the bleeding accidents of his Trojan War squaddies in 1200 BC.

•Description: this fragrant herb has foliage like fern and its name millefolium manner 1000 leaves because yarrow leaves are finely partitioned. The plant has an erect, angular

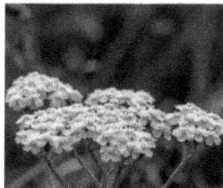

stem and lacy leaves that clasp beneath its easy stem. Its leaves can expand up to 6 inches tall.

eleven.Cleavers

•Scientific name: Gallium aparine

•Origin: This amusing herb is a weed that may be decided developing in fields throughout North America and Europe. Its nickname, bedstraw, occurred due to the fact the plant became used as bedding. It is thought Mary introduced cleavers to Jesus' manger. Being a plant in the coffee own family, cleaver seeds had been roasted and substituted as espresso in nearby Sweden.

•Description: This mountaineering weed has lengthy stalks and loopy leaves that without troubles fasten to other gadgets to facilitate the easy spreading of its seeds. It has been featured in traditional Chinese treatment, native Indian treatments and remains used in recent times as a diuretic.

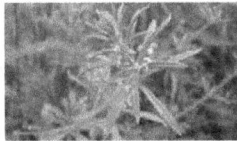

12.Gumweed

•Scientific call: Grindelia squarrosa

•Origin: this quick-lived plant is community to treasured and western North America which incorporates California, New Mexico, Texas, British Columbia, and Quebec.

•Description: The gumweed herb blooms from July to the quit of September producing many yellow ray vegetation. It may be determined growing in streamsides and roadsides. Gumweed has grey-inexperienced leaves and might broaden as much as forty

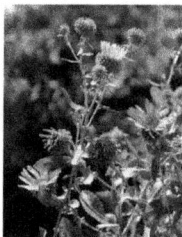

inches tall.

thirteen. Fennel

•Scientific name: Foeniculum vulgare

•Origin: fennel now grows plentifully in hundreds of elements of the arena however at the begin grew inside the Mediterranean vicinity. Its name is derived from the Latin word 'foeniculum' due to this little hay describing its feathery leaves. The name additionally refers to its conventional use in nurturing goats to reinforce the great of their milk.

•Description: This perennial herb is from the carrot own family. The flowery plant has feathery leaves and yellow vegetation. Fennel generally grows on dry soil near riverbanks and sea coasts. The great-smelling herb seems and tastes similar to the plant anise however the are very one-of-a-kind.

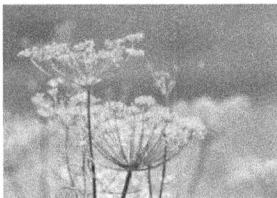

14.Mugwort

•Scientific name: Artemisia vulgaris

•Origin: this plant is indigenous to Asia and temperate Northern Europe however can be determined in plenty of regions of North America. Chinese songs from three BC factor out this ancient herb.

•Description: this daisy own family plant smells like sage, has sour leaves, and an angular stem. It generally grows as plenty as four ft however can effects climb to 6 toes. Its leaves are whitish underneath and darkish green above. In the summer season, mugwort blooms with a darkish orange or yellow plant life. The mugwort plant is a hard survivor, it could be discovered developing in the maximum now not probably of places.

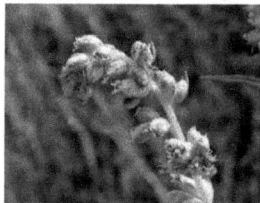

15. Mullein

•Scientific call: Verbascum thapsus

•Origin: the plant is indigenous to the Mediterranean, Asia, North Africa, and Europe. Today, it could be determined in lots of additives of Australia and North America. Its call is derived from the Latin phrase 'mollis' which means that mild. Since the leaves have a very soft texture, we are pronouncing that may be a befitting name.

•Description: the golden yellow vegetation of mullein are piled on a towering stalk in the course of open areas and fields anywhere within the international. An oil infusion may be gotten from the candy vegetation. The leaves and flowers may be used as a dye or perhaps the dried leaves aren't useless.

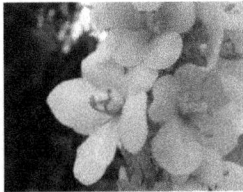

sixteen. Yellow Dock

•Scientific call: Rumex Crispus

•Origin: this herb is neighborhood to Western Asia and Europe but now grows at some point of North America. Many nearby American tribes used yellow dock appreciably for remedies from constipation to wound infection and yellow fever.

•Description: yellow dock has slender leaves that curl at the edges and fade away as they climb better up the stem. The flowers are a green seed that turns brownish or deep red within the fall indicating it's time for harvest.

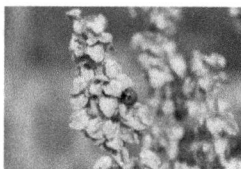

17.Parsley

•Scientific call: Petroselinum Crispus

•Origin: parsley is one of the maximum famous culinary herbs of all time. It originated from the Mediterranean areas of Tunisia, Algeria, and Southern Italy but is now notably grown throughout Europe and america. Greek mythology says parsley came from the blood of Archemorus, the forbearer of demise. This taste-improving, nutritious and medicinal meals became likely related to loss of life because it has an uncanny resemblance to 'fool's parsley', a poisonous plant additionally of Mediterranean starting region.

•Description: because parsley is inside the fennel and carrot family, it's far no wonder the roots are healthy to be eaten. The flavor of the foundation is bitter, now not candy however it is very nutritious. The curly leaves of the herb also are used as a meals garnish

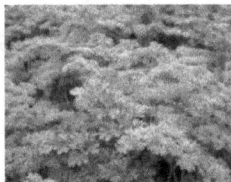

because it enhances the clean smooth appearance of a dish.

18.Chamomile

•Scientific call: Matricaria recutita

•Origin: chamomile originated in West Asia and Europe. From ancient instances, the medicinal developments of the herb were valued with the aid of Romans, Egyptians, and Greeks. Many cultures considered the herb a god-sent plant. The call is gotten from the Latin phrase 'matrix' which means womb. This refers to the soothing abilties it offers like that of a mom.

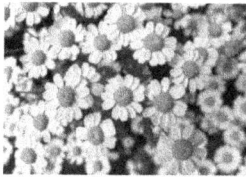

•Description: this agency of daisy-like flowery flora from the Asteraceae circle of relatives has been fed on for hundreds of years and most popularly as a tea. It is used to address a large shape of medical conditions but indigestion is the maximum famous.

19. Holy Basil

•Scientific name: Ocimum sanctum

•Origin: the aromatic perennial herb isn't always similar to the Thai herb plant normally used to taste soups. Holy basil is indigenous to India however has been extensively cultivated all over the tropics of Southeast Asia, West Africa, Australia, and some international locations within the Middle East. Ayurveda texts relationship once more to 1000 BC describe this leafy inexperienced plant as 'the incomparable one' and claim it's miles an embodiment of Tulasi, Lord Vishnu's consort.

•Description: holy basil is a small perennial shrub that can expand up to three.3 feet tall. It has a peppery quite spiced flavor and is considered a sacred plant in Hinduism. The leaves are generally purple or inexperienced with a hairy stem and easy leaves developing in opposite suggestions alongside the stalk.

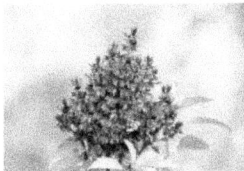

20. Fenugreek

•Scientific name: Trigonella foenum-graecum

•Origin: fenugreek is neighborhood to Western Asia, Southern Europe, and the larger Mediterranean vicinity. Now, it's miles usually cultivated in China, India, and the Middle East. In ancient times, fenugreek come to be utilized in Ayurvedic medicinal drug, Chinese treatment, and European people medicinal drug.

•Description: the leaves, twigs, roots, and seeds of fenugreek are beneficial whether or not or not or not dried or glowing. It has a cluster of 3 small obovate leaflets with a single stem much less than three ft tall. The plant has a sturdy aroma and grows erect.

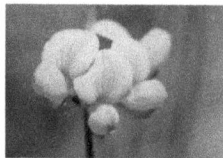

Whether you're a vegetarian, paleo dieter in any other case you eat quite lots a few factor, you could find out appropriate herbs for your preference of food. Make a addiction of eating herbs every day to enhance your health and growth the vitamins of each meal.

With so a whole lot of those herbs to be had, your flavor buds will not be jaded. If you grow your herbs sparkling or inventory up from your nearby farmers marketplace, you may enjoy the blessings of herbs all three hundred and sixty 5 days spherical. Some of these vegetation can even be dried or frozen to extend their shelf lifestyles.

Chapter 3: Benefits of Common Herbs

Industrial prescribed drugs and technological advancements have edged out effective potions and elixirs for surgical techniques and tablets when it comes to healthcare. Although this is the case, herbs have not misplaced their efficiency. People who need a more potent immune machine, large boosts in nutrients, and answers to diverse ailments even though choose natural treatments observed in herbs.

Many not unusual herbs can be implemented for recuperation and medicinal functions. Take a glance underneath at how the normal herbs you're to be had touch with every day can be beneficial to you and your properly-being.

1.Burdock

Burdock has been an active element in traditional Chinese treatment for loads of years. Originally, it come to be normally used to cope with digestive and diuretic issues however modern-day-day-day research has positioned many feasible uses for the herb.

•Skin conditions: while topically carried out to the pores and skin, the antibacterial houses in burdock permits combat pores and pores and pores and skin conditions like pimples, eczema, and psoriasis.

•Toxin removal: the herb is strong in using the bloodstream of toxins. Burdock can detoxify the blood and sell higher move.

•Antioxidants: burdock houses numerous remarkable antioxidants which incorporates luteolin, phenolic acids, and quercetin.

2.Calendula

There is factor out of calendula being applied in ancient Chinese and Ayurvedic treatment. The sunny blooms of calendula are effective as a wound recovery, anti-inflammatory, antimicrobial herb to treatment all way of skin issues.

•Skin recuperation: oil can be extracted from the calendula flower for topical use in treating wounds, sunburns, bruises, rashes, stings, and bug bites. You also can make a salve from the herb and use it to treat eczema, acne, swellings, and cold sores. It can also be used on cervical dysplasia and yeast infections.

•Other blessings: the herb is in shape to be eaten and can be utilized in meals, salads, and tea as a calming thing. A yellow dye may be extracted from the vegetation and used on food or fabric.

3.Chickweed

In ancient instances, the leaves, plant life, and stem of chickweed have been used teas, extracts, and decorations. The effective plant additives on this herb are the cause for its blessings.

•Skin situations: even as rubbed topically, chickweed can cope with itchy pores and pores and skin, rashes, wounds, burns, touch dermatitis, eczema, and psoriasis. It may also additionally also be used towards nappy rash in infants.

•Weight loss: while nicely administered, chickweed may moreover want to assist fight weight troubles-delivered about via progesterone.

four.Dandelion

This herb is a pesky weed for max human beings but nearby Americans and historical Chinese healers used dandelion to cope with liver and stomach conditions. Dandelion root, smooth or dried, may be used to make tinctures, teas, and poultices.

•Skin harm: dandelion can be dried, floor, and made proper into a paste through together with some water. This soothes pores and pores and skin problems like eczema, acne, rashes, psoriasis, and boils. Its antipruritic and anti-inflammatory features can also assist save you sun damage.

•Liver damage: even as consumed as a tonic, dandelion cleanses the liver, relieving it of strain and makes room for liver regeneration.

•Blood pressure: research shows that the diuretic effects of dandelion can be useful in treating premenstrual bloating, prediabetes, and water retention.

five.Echinacea

The red coneflower isn't famous for no purpose. This herb is packed complete of benefits recognize to fight issues of contamination, pain, flu, migraines, and others.

•Skin issues: the anti-bacterial and anti inflammatory houses of echinacea limit the increase of Propionibacterium, acne-inflicting bacteria. When carried out topically, echinacea moreover allows reduce wrinkles, hydrate pores and pores and pores and skin, and enhance the signs and symptoms and symptoms of eczema.

•Cancer: this herb is useful in suppressing the increase of most cancers cells and possibly triggers the lack of lifestyles of cancer cells too.

•Reduces anxiety: echinacea includes caffeic acid, rosmarinic, and alkamides which might be all useful in combating tension.

6.Elderflower

Although elderflower is extra notably used for its flavoring, the herb has many medicinal benefits. Elderflower has antioxidant, anti inflammatory, anti-most cancers, and antimicrobial homes useful for preventing ailments.

•Respiratory illnesses: the anti inflammatory and antiseptic homes of elderflower make it pleasant for preventing the flu, sinus infections, colds, and one-of-a-kind respiratory illnesses.

•Laxative and diuretic: elderflower can help ease constipation.

•Boost immune system: its antiviral and antibacterial houses are useful for combating allergies and boosting the immune device.

•Wounds: it may be used to save you bleeding from injuries.

•Blood sugar: elderflower can artwork like insulin to lessen blood sugar stages.

7.Nettle

Stinging nettle has been useful for herbal remedies thinking about the reality that ancient instances. Roman soldiers massaged it into their pores and pores and skin to hold warm temperature and Egyptians used it to address back ache and arthritis. Nettle has many nutrients at the side of nutrition A, severa B nutrients, vitamins C, and K, all of the important amino acids, sodium, iron, calcium, and more.

•Reduce infection: the herb has houses that would help your body fight infection.

•Hay fever: nettle suggests quite some promise for treating hay fever. It stops inflammations that reason allergic reactions.

•Controls blood sugar: nettle is hooked up to lowering blood sugar in humans and animals alike.

eight.Oats

Oats are a gluten-free superfood wealthy with minerals, nutrients, antioxidants, and fiber. The plant has been cultivated for medicinal treatments lengthy before it became grown as a meals.

•Contains beta-glucan: this fiber is useful for decreasing blood sugar tiers, reducing cholesterol, growing pinnacle micro organism, and making you experience fuller for longer.

•Protects from ldl ldl cholesterol harm: due to the immoderate amount of beta-glucan in oats, ldl ldl cholesterol go with the flow is decreased on your body whilst you eat oats.

•Weight loss: due to the truth oats are very filling, it can help with weight reduction in the end.

•Skincare: finely ground oats help shield the pores and skin, cope with itching, and reduce inflammation.

9.Peppermint

Romans, Greeks, and Egyptians used peppermint for remedy centuries in the beyond. You can use the herb as an extract, a tea, or an oil.

•Relieves stomach disillusioned: doctors endorse peppermint for alleviating nausea and vomiting in addition to unique belly discomforts.

•Irritable bowel symptoms and symptoms: peppermint pills are used to deal with constipation, gas, and diarrhea.

•Headache: the menthol in peppermint can reduce migraines and headaches.

•Mouth germs: peppermint is referred to as a breath freshener and its antibacterial homes assist to kill the deliver of terrible breath too.

•Energy improve: peppermint oil can chase sleep and dullness away to offer you a lift in some unspecified time in the future of artwork.

10.Yarrow

From the time of the Trojan War, this daisy herb has now not been forgotten.

•Toothache: chewing the sparkling leaves of yarrow herb has been recognised to reduce toothache.

•Healing effect: yarrow oil is infused in shampoos and other merchandise to result in a chilled, restoration effect.

•Wound bleeding: yarrow promotes sweating to halt bleeding from wounds. It is even used to alleviate heavy bleeding from menstrual cycles.

11.Cleavers

From historic times, cleavers has acted as a diuretic in herbal remedy. It has been used to address bladder infections with the resource of selling urine and relieving edema. The aerial factors of cleaver herb are used by current-day herbalists to:

•Support the lymphatic glands. Taking cleavers promotes herbal cleansing of the body.

•Support mucosal membrane fitness of the pores and skin and urinary tracts.

12.Gumweed

This herb is a excellent herbal muscle relaxant. Favored for its medicinal tendencies by using the usage of many tribes of Native Americans, gumweed is commonly used to treat bronchial troubles and bronchial asthma.

•Lung troubles: this herb permits to loosen up and open your airlines to alleviate problems like bronchial allergies and bronchitis. It furthermore permits do away with phlegm and catarrh just so breathing is progressed.

•Calming: gumweed reduces the reactivity of nerve endings internal your bronchial tube really so the coronary coronary heart price is decreased and the character is calmed.

•Skin issues: at the same time as used as a topical remedy, gumweed can deal with problems like burns, boils, poison ivy rash, insect bites, and dermatitis.

13.Fennel

The bulb of the fennel plant has a licorice taste however this taste is stronger inside the seed because it includes a few oil. Aside from the culinary uses of fennel, the herb has many fitness blessings you may experience.

•Reduce menstrual pain: girls who take fennel extracts each day experience a whole lot tons much less menstrual cramps than women who don't.

•Weight manipulate: fennel makes you experience fuller without inclusive of greater calories. It moreover lets in mystery anethole to help with appetite manage.

•Relieves constipation: many cultures use fennel as a laxative to ease the passing of stool during constipation.

14. Mugwort

Because the mugwort plant grows aggressively and can take over entire areas in a quick even as, human beings cope with and damage it as a weed. However, mugwort is thought to reduce itching, sell blood go with the glide, increase electricity, and assist a healthy liver.

•Diuretic: it offers with fluid retention via growing a person's urine output.

•Better menstrual cycles: it acts as an emmenagogue and promotes ordinary, uniform menstrual cycles.

•Calms nerves: is substantially used as a nervine.

•Others: mugwort is implemented in treating numerous fitness problems along with colic, fatigue, epilepsy, headache, constipation, vomiting, hypochondria, and restlessness.

15.Mullein

Some compounds observed in the plants and leaves of this herb act as expectorants or demulcents. Because of this, mullein can calm pores and skin inflammations and irritations of a few inner factors.

•Ear infections: while used as an lively detail in eardrops, mullein is strong in managing ear ache and otalgia.

•Flu: mullein attacks viruses that cause the flu and prevent vital illnesses that rise up from the flu consisting of pneumonia.

•Others: herbalists additionally make use of mullein in treating coughs, allergies, bronchitis, and infections in the top breathing tract.

sixteen. Yellow dock

Yellow dock is a exceptional herb for present day-day herbal treatments. Among many makes use of, it's miles useful in liver cleansing and healthful digestion.

•Blood detoxing: it's miles used for cleaning and detoxifying the blood.

•Diarrhea: eating yellow dock is a famous remedy for malaria and diarrhea.

•Fever: the herb is loaded with manganese, nutrients A and phosphorus, all powerful medication for fever.

•Anemia: because of the fact yellow dock cleanses the blood, it is been used to heal anemia.

•Throat problems: the yellow dock is popularly acknowledged for its sore throat and intestine treating homes.

17.Parsley

Parsley isn't always your normal garnish. The herb includes iron, calcium, vitamins C, weight-reduction plan K, and plenty of antioxidant compounds beneficial preventing numerous illnesses.

•Allergies: you could extract essential oils from parsley leaves to help address seasonal hypersensitive reactions with the useful resource of the usage of suppressing contamination.

•Diabetes: it was decided that parsley is powerful in tackling liver harm as a result of diabetes. The herb is entire of antioxidants that make it sturdy enough to fight diabetes.

•Breast cancer: parsley produces apigenin, a non-toxic chemical for treating most cancers. Apigenin is known for decreasing the tumor period of aggressive breast cancer.

18.Chamomile

Chamomile can be very famous as an useful resource for sleep but it's far beneficial for coping with tension too.

•Anxiety: clinical trials with chamomile suggest it has diffused anti-tension results on people laid low with tension issues.

•Insomnia: delivered to its anti-anxiety houses, chamomile is likewise a moderate sedative that could result in sleep while administered within the proper amount.

•Digestive troubles: chamomile stops the growth of belly ulcer-causing bacteria. It is also beneficial for decreasing stomach muscle spasms.

•Oral health: the anti inflammatory and antimicrobial houses of chamomile make it effective in competition to plaque and gingivitis while used as a mouthwash.

19. Holy Basil

This medicinal herb packs quite a few fitness-boosting outcomes together with anti-inflammatory, antimicrobial, antioxidant, antidiarrheal, anticoagulant, anti-diabetic, anti-arthritic, and more.

•Chronic infection: the Ayurvedic exercise of consuming a excessive quality quantity of holy basil every day has been tested to assist fight a gaggle of gift-day persistent diseases.

•Inflammation: many studies have pointed to holy basil as an powerful device in competition to severa ailments related to infection. The herb can work on my own or with different substances to restrict inflammation.

•Other applications: holy basil has many different medicinal advantages including the treatment of pressure, tension, fever, decrease lower back pain, ringworm, malaria, dysentery, bronchial bronchial asthma, snakebites, and coronary heart illness.

20. Fenugreek

Although fenugreek seeds are bitter, this plant may be used towards a group of scientific issues.

•Diabetes: the chemical substances and fiber contained in fenugreek slow the absorption of carbohydrates and sugar. This will boom the body's insulin degree.

•Boost fertility: men who often take fenugreek experienced a boost in testosterone, libido, and strength.

•Prevent cancer: the plant includes phytochemicals beneficial in stopping cancers.

•Aid nursing moms: Ayurvedic remedy recommends fenugreek to growth milk outstanding in breastfeeding mothers.

Take word that this isn't always an exhaustive listing, now not even near. Each medicinal property of every herb cited above may be very real and may usually be boosted by means of the use of manner of combining herbs. Blends of herbs can shape ointments, teas, and tinctures with expanded healing functionality on your body. Always make sure to apply natural merchandise which might be homegrown or furnished from dependable belongings. This ensures the nice of your surrender products and ensures effectiveness. Also, be sure to attempting to find advice from your healthcare expert earlier than concocting herb combos for non-public remedy.

Chapter 4: Tea Recipes

As a species, human beings frequently make certain to cook dinner with herbs, but, utilizing them in refreshments may be similarly as carrying out. Other than having surprising aromas, the therapeutic houses of herbs are in a few instances intensified with the growth of boiling water.

An collection of herbal tea mixes is obtainable for buying, but frequently the ones business corporation mixes hire faux flavorings and are not the actual piece thru any stretch of the creativeness. You can preserve an amazing distance from those through making your own mixes making use of characteristic flowers and herbs you have were given got grown or amassed yourself. Blending your herbs for tea is as clean as choosing the fragrances that intrigue you and combining up your preferred choices. In summer time, you could choice a delicious frosted tea, at the equal time as wintry climate can also additionally see you fermenting a first rate warm temperature tea to keep away from the relax.

First of all, herbal tea can also help conflict colds by way of way of clearing nasal entries and halting huge hacks. This is furthermore stated to reduce bronchial bronchial asthma. Herbal tea is understood to help assimilation/digestion. It can assist split down fat and boost up the purging of the belly, an outstanding way to lessen the thing effects of swelling, acid reflux sickness, and heaving. The extraordinary teas for this are dandelion, peppermint, ginger, and chamomile. Herbal tea consists of most cancers prevention sellers that could deliver down the risk of ceaseless contamination. The high-quality teas for this are echinacea, ginger, elderberry, and yarrow root. Here are some of the tea recipes which you can effortlessly put together at home.

Hot Burdock Tea

Due to its medicinal houses, Burdock Herb, scientifically known as, Artium lappa, may be with out issues made into tea. It can every be sliced or immediately be added to soups and broths. Initially, it became used merely as a medicinal herb and have been effective in curing, measles, bloodless, sore throat, arthritis, and masses of different common ailments like tonsillitis, and plenty of others. But now the National Institute of Health within the USA has these days claimed that Burdock might also additionally have useful consequences on human fitness. Recent studies display that Burdock also can have a remedy for HIV, bacterial infections, maximum cancers, and kidney stones. But ensure to consult health care experts earlier than the use of any form of herb as a eternal medication.

Ingredients:

•2 cups of water

•Fresh or dried burdock root

•Stainless-metal teapot

Procedure:

i.First, select a sparkling burdock root. Keep in mind that those will no longer stay easy for lengthy and often will begin to rot. So, if there are some leftover Burdock roots, you can upload them to some curry or soup.

ii. In case you have got were given determined on a merely glowing root you can certainly wipe the dust with a clean material. On the opposite hand, if you have picked a piece older root you could smooth the burdock root thru scrapping off the edges with a knife.

iii.In case you don't have a easy root, you can additionally use a tablespoon of dried burdock root powder.

iv.Add calmly chopped portions of the foundation to the teapot and add 3 to four cups of filtered water. Heat very well until the water boils and then lower the warmth to permit it constantly cook dinner dinner on low warmness for as a minimum 2 to half-hour. This will extract out all the essence of the herb.

v. Serve the tea warm. You can keep and consume the tea as a detox at a few degree inside the day. But keep in mind that burdock is a diuretic so do not over-eat.

Fresh Calendula Tea

Calendula is likewise an ancient herb and is frequently used in tea. Due to its giant makes use of, the herb will be very famous and is quite well-known for its therapeutic use. The tea may be implemented as a gargle for sore throat. It also can be used as an anti-inflammatory agent and may be implemented to ruptured pores and skin. You can without issues wash your face for its anti-acne houses. Pouring a few on the foot may also moreover remedy athletes' foot. Or it may additionally be used as a rinsing agent if you have itchy eyes. While most of those are the outdoor makes use of of the tea, it is also recommended to have cured gastric ulcers and sore throat. It can also assist ruin a immoderate fever via sweating. But you need to are searching for advice from your scientific doctor earlier than the use of it as any kind of right remedy when you have persistent situations because of the fact it is able to additionally accentuate bleeding in menstruation and pregnant women must are seeking recommendation from their gynecologists first.

Ingredients

•2 – three Cups of freshwater.

•Fresh Calendula Flowers

•Stainless-steel teapot

Procedure

i.If you have got were given were given picked it glowing, then you may actually upload the flowers to the teapot after washing them with tap water and maintain on with the following step. In the case of dried flora, mash dried flowers and grind them.

ii. Add 1 to 2 tablespoons of the mashed calendula powder to the teapot.

iii.Add three to four cups of freshwater to the teapot.

iv.Cover the pot and allow the water boil.

v. After boiling, go away the pot on low warm temperature to extract all the aroma of the herb. This will make the tea more centered. If you want to maintain it slight. Just pull it off a chunk earlier.

vi.Serve it warm. Or you could definitely permit infuse till it cools down. You can preserve it and devour it at a few degree inside the day.

Chickweed Herbal Tea

Chickweed tea has been carried out as a domestic-grown remedy due to the truth the 16th century supporting with breathing problems in addition to pores and skin maladies and aggravations. This tea (to be taken in) can be prescribed to human beings with bad assimilation or maybe to the ones experiencing tuberculosis. The chickweed herb carries various vitamins and minerals. It is rich in Vitamin B, B-complicated, A, and C. It additionally includes calcium, zinc, potassium, flavonoids, and iron collectively with many other vitamins. All the ones important vitamins and minerals make this a wholesome beverage to be included to your weekly healthy dietweight-reduction plan. It can therapy skin and tissue troubles, can act as a blood cleaner, help you in dropping weight, and be used as a natural sedative.

Ingredients:

• 2 to a few cups of water

• The aerial part of chickweed plant

• Stainless-steel teapot

Procedure:

i.This recipe will start through way of boiling water within the teapot. Start heating 2 to three cups of water till it boils.

ii. Now we can add the chickweed herb to the cups. If you've got were given dried chickweed, upload 1 tablespoon to the cups.

In case you have got were given clean herb then add 2 tablespoons to every cup.

iii.If you have got taken sparkling herb, then consider to lessen the leaves to permit the flavor out.

iv.Once the water has boiled, upload it warm into the cups and permit the herb steep for 5 to 10 mins.

v.   You also can upload honey to the tea to even enhance the taste.

vi.Serve it warm.

Dandelion Tea

Many people realise dandelion as a outside weed, however if you have a study its fitness benefits it proves to be a totally useful flower. Dandelion tea might also moreover have many powerful effects for your digestive tool. It improves urge for meals and soothes digestive ailments. It moreover remedy alternatives the cleaning of the liver. Dandelion tea acts as a herbal diuretic and might flush out extra fluid from the frame. Moreover, the tea is complete of masses of antioxidants that prevent the frame from all varieties of cellular damage and keeps the frame and pores and pores and pores and skin easy.

Ingredients

•2 – 3 cups of water

•Fresh dandelion plants

•2-three Tablespoon of dried stevia leaf

•3-4 limes (juiced)

Procedure

i.The first step is to choose smooth dandelions. Pick first-rate yellow components of the flower and pull off any more leaves which can be later utilized in salads and so forth.

ii. Wash/Rinse with bloodless water very well.

iii.Take the water in the stainless steel pot and start to warm temperature. Heat till the water boils.

iv.Add dandelion plant life to the boiling water. Cover the lid and allow the taste steep for 15 to twenty minutes.

v. Add lime juice and stir properly.

vi.Serve it bloodless or at room temperature.

vii. You also can shop it to use at some point of the day.

Mint - Echinacea Tea

Echinacea tea is a domestic-grown beverage most generally produced the usage of the Echinacea purpura plant. Echinacea is a famous solution for influenza, colds, and plenty of great illnesses. A few human beings moreover be given that echinacea can lessen torment, stop malignancy, decorate intellectual properly-being, and decrease quite some skin troubles. In any case, mainstream researchers and medical doctors do not consider to the advantages of echinacea tea and a few have communicated problems for echinacea signs and signs and signs. The flavor of echinacea tea is frequently portrayed as tongue-shivering. Truth be recommended, a few domestic-grown item producers view this awesome as proof of the herb's adequacy. Echinacea is normally joined with mint or with specific fixings, for example, lemongrass to make an more and more lovely tasting tea.

Ingredients

•2 – 3 cups of water

•Dried echinacea leaves

•1 tsp lemongrass (dried)

•1 tsp mint (dried)

Instructions

i.Grind the materials and mix the three.

ii. Add water to the heating teapot and allow it boil.

iii.Add all the combined herbs inside the boiling water.

iv.Allow the aggregate to settle as it will steep for about 15 minutes. This will help the flavor ooze out and blend in water.

v. Enjoy simple or with honey. You can also enhance the taste thru along with awesome sweeteners.

Elderflower Tea

It is a shame that elderflower tea isn't broadly recognized but for the reason that this natural tea is exceedingly precious. Additionally, it's miles heavenly in taste, and easy. Elderflower tea has a whole lot of advantages. It is also stated to encompass immoderate degrees of a couple of vitamins. Most not unusual of it truly is Vit C, due to which it could act as a effective antioxidant. The herb is supposed to reinforce the coronary coronary heart and the immune device. Elderflower does help the metabolism and calms the belly. It can also soothe stomach cramps. Additionally, it purifies the blood and moreover stimulates kidney activity.

Ingredients:

• 2 – 3 Cups of Fresh Water

• Elderflower (Dried or Fresh)

• Stainless – metal teapot.

Procedure:

i.To make elderflower tea from sparkling or dried elderflowers really pick out a few flower bunches of the clean plant. If you have have been given dried leaves, you may grind them to apply in the subsequent step.

ii.   If taking glowing flowers you want to carefully reduce all of the stems as they may be now not regular to consume. They may be poisonous.

iii.Fill the teapot with water and set it to warmth, till it boils.

iv. Place the flower petals or 1 teaspoon of dried powder within the cup and pour the latest water.

v. Cover the lid and allow the combination be given 15 to twenty minutes.

vi. Enjoy your glowing pot of elderflower tea. You also can add honey for similarly sweetening.

Nettle Herb Tea

Nettle is a shrub that is mainly observed in Europe and Asia. Scientifically known as Urtica dioica, nettle shrub has a number of medicinal houses and can be used as natural remedy. You may want to make it proper right into a tea, which now not only tastes proper but also can remedy urinal tract infections similarly to being a scrumptious additive for your soups. Moreover, Nettle shrub has been used considerably for curing arthritis ache and sore muscle companies, Some research had been completed lower back in 2013, display that nettle leaf extract lowers the blood sugar tiers in kind 2 diabetic humans. Recipe for making scrumptious Nettle tea is as follows:

Ingredients:

•2 - 3 cups of consuming water

•Nettle leaves (sparkling or dries powder)

•Stainless-metallic teapot

Procedure:

i.Add water to the teapot and set it to warmth.

ii. Add 2 to a few nettle leaves or 1 tablespoon nettle leaf powder when you have dry powder.

iii.Let the aggregate warmth for 15 to 20 mins on low flame.

iv.When the water is ready to boil, flip off the range and allow it take a seat for five to 10 mins.

v. Add honey to the cups for sweetening the tea. You can also upload cinnamon or stevia for assed flavors.

Oats Tea

Oats are rich in solvent filaments which help in bringing down levels of cholesterol. These dissolvable strands assist increment intestinal adventure time and reduce glucose ingestion. Oats furthermore encompass beta-glucan which is a lipid bringing down the operator. Oats can also serve to be a completely sturdy breakfast opportunity. Be it a handy answer for cravings for meals, moderate, and wholesome night time nibble or sturdy electricity offering substance that allows you via your rushed morning, oats are actually the one superfood that may sincerely meet itself to fit your requirements. Oat teas have all the essential vitamins you probable can encompass in a balanced eating regimen.

Ingredients:

•2 – three cups of water.

• 2 TB rolled oats

• 1 cinnamon stick

• Honey (greater or a whole lot an awful lot less to taste)

• 2 tsp natural vanilla extract (extra or a extraordinary deal a great deal less to flavor)

Procedure:

i. Take a saucepan and positioned 2 to three cups of water in it.

ii. Put oats, cinnamon stick, into the saucepan and bring as a whole lot as a boil.

iii. Turn the warmth down and cover the lid for approximately half of-hour.

iv. Turn off warmness and upload honey and vanilla.

v. Strain to take away oats if desired.

vi. Serve heat.

Peppermint Tea

Peppermint frames a giant piece of our lives; from giving our irritated stomach a few help to giving our liquids an invigorating taste and fragrance. Its calmative houses can leave you genuinely comfortable, and in intellectual peace. You can also have said about peppermint tea that makes for a super flavor and having giant health and beauty benefits. Some peppermint teas will let you lessen weight. It additionally permits in relieving stomach acidity, lessens acid reflux disorder disease, makes your pores and pores and skin gleam, initiates rest, and offers satiety, further assisting you to get in form. There is scarcely any symptom of peppermint tea; so, you can drink it on every occasion you want to.

Ingredients:

• 2 to a few tablespoon beaten (glowing) peppermint leaves or dried leaves

• three – four cups of eating water.

• Stainless-metal Pots

Procedure:

i.The first step is to select out glowing leaves. Crush the leaves to make it effortlessly mixable.

ii. Wash/Rinse with cold water thoroughly.

iii.Take the water inside the chrome steel pot and start to warm temperature. Heat until the water boils.

iv.Add the beaten peppermint leaves to the boiling water. Cover the lid and permit the flavor steep for 15 to twenty mins.

v. Add lime juice and stir nicely.

vi.Serve it hot, cold, or at room temperature.

vii. You also can shop it to use at a few stage within the day.

Yarrow Tea

Yarrow is a long-stemmed member of the sunflower family. Yarrow tea may additionally need to have many brilliant outcomes for your digestive tool. It improves urge for food and soothes digestive ailments. It also remedies menstrual problems. Yarrow tea acts as a natural diuretic and may flush out more fluid from the frame and additionally fights micro organism, helping your immune gadget to live robust. Moreover, the tea is packed with hundreds of antioxidants that save you the body from all kinds of cell damage and maintains the frame and pores and skin clean.

Ingredients

•2 – 3 cups of water

•Fresh Yarrow plant life

•3-four limes (juiced)

Procedure

i.The first step is to select sparkling Yarrow. Pick best white elements of the flower and pull off any extra leaves.

ii. Wash/Rinse with cold water thoroughly.

iii.Take the water in the stainless-steel pot and begin to warm temperature. Heat till the water boils.

iv.Add Yarrow plants to the boiling water. Cover the lid and allow the taste steep for 15 to twenty mins.

v. Add lime juice and stir properly.

vi.Serve it cold or at room temperature.

vii. You can also shop it to apply at some point of the day.

Chapter 5: Making Your Own Tinctures
What Is A Tincture?

The universe of flowers is an fantastic one. There is an abundance of segments in plant life that serve to make sure them at exceptional levels of innovation, as there are this form of exceptional kind of forces at play

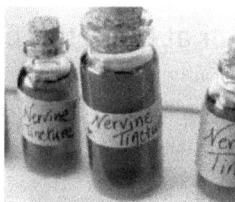

inclusive of weather, predators (counting us), and soil superb. At the issue at the same time as we deplete the ones plant materials in exclusive structures, we are able to likewise get hold of the rewards – but, figuring out a manner to set up those flora and herbs successfully isimportant.. This is the area hand made tinctures and tonics are to be had in.

For quite a long term, herbalists have been growing combos of tinctures to repair normal ailments. Regardless of whether or no longer or now not you need help within the digestive gadget, relaxation, or a stimulating enhance to start your day, there is probably a herb that can help. Herbs can be applied dried or glowing to make tinctures. Fresh herbs have a greater grounded perfume, however are not as effective as dried herbs. Fresh herbs can upload an aroma to the tincture, however dried herbs are clinically more beneficial.

Tinctures make it simple to consume the regular immunity-boosting materials discovered in wonderful flora. They are commonly moderately brief to make and may be successfully prepared at home. The availability of natural recovery processes like tinctures is most in all likelihood a extensive motivation in the again of why an expected 80 percentage of the total population is based upon on the ones drug remedies for a trouble in their fitness desires. Tinctures are clean to make and are as useful as another natural tea. At the factor at the identical time as you need a spark off response, as an example, herbs for fast rest, a tincture may come up with an increasing number of brief results. For nutritive herbs which could take a hint even as of intake to get outcomes, every a tincture or a tea is probably first-rate. It all relies upon

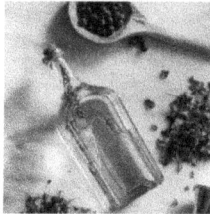

on one's man or woman preference. Some commonly regarded Tinctures which may be actually made at home are defined.

A tincture is simplest a centered herbal combination made with liquor, which may be taken straight or diluted in tea or water. So, it's miles a few one-of-a-kind technique of having rid of the dynamic factors from a herb, with the exception that you are the usage of alcohol in preference to vinegar, water, or some different dissolvable. Due to the alcohol in tinctures, the extracts of the herbs quite actually take in into the blood and the consequences are visible inner an hour. Due to their lively assimilation, tinctures display to be the satisfactory treatment for things like belly issues, pain, anxiety, and precise sleep-related issues. Commonly people hire tinctures for the following sicknesses.

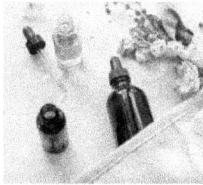

•Stress/tension

•Cold/flu

•Indigestion

•Allergies

•Insomnia

Ingredients Required For Tinctures

It is rather easy to make tinctures at home, the use of the herb of your desire. Tinctures, as effective as they may be, may be made very quickly. You probable can't inform for positive whether or now not or not the tinctures are real or now not in case you are shopping for them from a close-by herbal shop. It is normally higher to steer them to on your kitchen. Here is a full-size list of objects that you will be seeking to make tinctures at domestic.

- Alcohol

- eighty proof alcohol

80 evidence alcohol is taken into consideration a favored for maximum tinctures. This form of Alcohols (eighty proof Vodka) may be used on herbs that don't have a whole lot moisture content material material. Some of those herbs are fennel, thyme, bay, dill, and so on.

- eighty evidence alcohol + 100 ninety evidence grain alcohol

A aggregate within the ratio (1:1) of eighty evidence Alcohol and a hundred 90 proof alcohol may be used to extract the substances from extra risky plant additives because it has a better alcohol content cloth cloth. This may be used for herbs with better moisture content. Some of these herbs encompass parsley, cilantro, sage, oregano, and so forth.

• one hundred ninety proof grain alcohol

a hundred 90 proof grain alcohol is generally used for dissolving thick plant quantities inclusive of resins and gums. These are discovered within the dried plant topics similar to the bark of timber, and so forth. While it makes tinctures, which can be strong in flavor, it may additionally extract essential aromatics and oils in flora. It can by some means dehydrate the tincture, which may have an impact at the prolonged-term first rate of the tincture.

Alternative To Alcohol

If you do no longer have get admission to to alcohol or because of some precise constraints, you are unable to utilize alcohol, you can as an opportunity use fireplace cider vinegar or food-grade glycerin. The distinction is that it'll then be known as an extract in desire to a tincture. This is an change approach but serves the same characteristic.

Herbs

Tinctures may be made with every, sparkling and dried herbs. You may additionally additionally even use leaves, flowers, and berries to do the identical. It is typically extremely good to apply glowing herbs for tinctures as it will final longer and can furthermore have huge prolonged-time period results.

No doubt, sparkling herbs serves excellent for tinctures but are not with no trouble available anywhere. Dried herbs are handiest to seek out because they closing longer and do now not rot without issues.

Some of the most commonplace herbs used for tincture nowadays are:

•Nettle

•Echinacea

•Licorice

•Elderberries

Instructions to make Tinctures

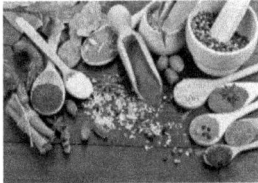

Step 01

Take a pint-sized glass jar with a lid. You can also additionally use a chunk of parchment or a plastic wrap. So, if you are the use of a jar with a metallic lid than take hold of that piece

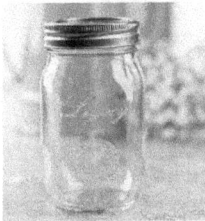

of plastic too. Find a nook of a room wherein this box can relaxation with out a top notch deal disturbance.

Step 02

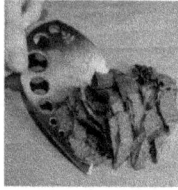

Take a pestle or a mortar and finely chop your herbs. You want to reduce them great enough to healthful the glass jar. Chopping the herbs offers them a large floor vicinity to dissolve the liquid, that you can add later. You also can toss the herbs without delay into the jar without reducing them however then the energy of the tincture is probably

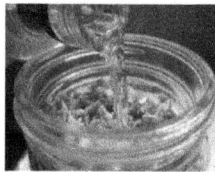

compromised.

Step 03

Once you're completed with Step 02, crammed the rest of the jar with Alcohol. Remember to fill the jar because of the reality whatever popping out above the liquid will begin to mold. Make sure that the ranges of liquid are an inch better than your herbs. So, to preserve the herbs from molding, submerge them well underneath the liquid ground.

Step 04

Screw on the lid tightly. If you are using a jar with a metal lid, then you will want to wrap the mouth of the jar with a piece of plastic wrap. After wrapping the piece over the mouth, screw the lid and location the jar in a cupboard. Remember to maintain the jar in a dry, cool, and dark vicinity truly so the extraction technique must with out issues

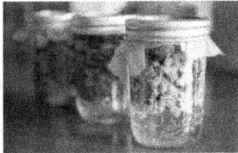

begin.

Step 05

Check at the jar each couple of days. Shake the jar now after which just so the herbs may additionally modify their positions to make the extraction way extra effective. Also, take a look at to look if the alcohol hasn't evaporated an excessive amount of. If you

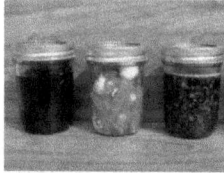

revel in that the herbs aren't submerged, then top it off with the same alcohol. Keep on checking the jar frequently for almost eight weeks.

Step 06

After the extraction way is whole, take an amber dropper bottle. Remember to take the bottle with a first rate-mesh strainer. Put the funnel inside the amber bottle and pour all the liquid from the jar into the funnel. This will pressure out all the herbs. To extract the final part of the tincture, take a cheesecloth and wrap the closing herbs within the material. Squeeze the cheesecloth to extract the stays thoroughly.

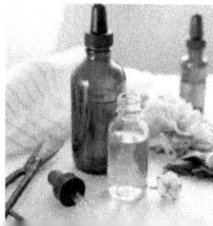

Step 07

If you have made multiple tinctures, then make certain you label them properly. When

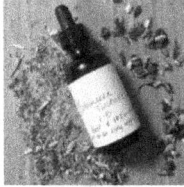

labeling the bottle write

•Herbs used

•Percent and Type of Alcohol

•Date and Time

This is it; you're organized along side your tincture. You need to make a tincture the usage of the herbs of your liking. The advantages of each herb are explained in the previous chapters.

How To Use The Tincture

To utilize this tincture, you could use different strategies.

1. You can constantly area some drops right

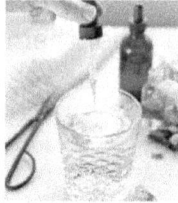

away beneath your tongue.

2. You can typically upload a few drops to a tumbler of water or a cup of tea.

The quantity of the tincture you are adding to the tea or water usually relies upon at the strength of the tincture. It additionally is based upon on the herbs used because of the truth some herbs are stronger than others. Your frame chemistry moreover impacts the quantity of tincture you may want to use.

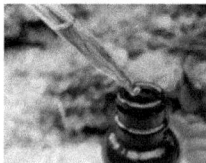

Most humans find it irresistible light however a few choose it strong.

Chapter 6: Grow Your Own

There's continuously this great, calming feeling about someone interacting with nature on a personal level. It is hard to apprehend why not greater human beings engage in developing their personal produce while it's so easy and a laugh; plus, you get to keep coins as fast as your little creations have matured and you can harvest them. So permit's attempt growing those herbs proper now!

Here's what you'll need to do:

Deciding Where to Grow

You'll should figure out which is extra great to you; both growing indoors (the use of containers) or developing outdoors. Objects which could damage your plants or tamper with ordinary growth are sturdy enforcers here. The trouble can be the canine out of doors or the kid internal; it's crucial to recognize which location is most secure and can be most type to your plant.

It's great to maintain in mind that a few herbs may additionally have a tougher time growing in bins due to the truth their root systems require sufficient region; herbs like horseradish, fennel, and lovage are some of the ones herbs at the identical time as many others can develop perfectly best in packing containers; the ones are like mint, chives, sage, bay, horehound, and wintry weather savory. Knowing this, a subject is probably a splendid start to your seedling to mature, but a few herbs can also need to be plotted on prepared earth to broaden nicely in the end.

Deciding Method of Growing

1.From Seeds

Acquiring seeds of the ideal herb you require from a store or a mature plant and appending an environment to it in case you want to stimulate the germination of the seed is needed here. Various seeds of herbs have particular goals and gestation durations and so obtaining information about this earlier than intending with propagation is critical or the seed might also additionally need to fail to germinate. Generally, most seeds of herbs germinate in temperatures approximated to 21°C with enough moisture supply and can take from consistent with week to 4 weeks in advance than they sprout seedlings.

(Tip: Placing the seeds internal a closed plastic bag and misting the innards with water can

make certain that there's enough humidity wished for germination of the seeds.)

2.From Seedlings

If lucky enough to already have seedlings of a herb, then preparations for propagation can begin at once thru placing the seedlings in plotted areas on prepared earth.

three.From Stem cuttings

It is possible to broaden a herb with the aid of way of reducing a part of the stem of a mature plant and setting it in water. Eventually, the stem reducing will grow roots and also you'll be capable of place it in the soil for similarly propagation.

Of direction, it might be great if every reducing of a positive herb must preserve to propagate and so developing top-rated situations (obtaining cuttings on the equal time as herbs are going thru sparkling growth like after harvesting or inside the course of the spring proper right here there can be multiplied growth of foliage) is vital for better achievement costs

Preparing the Environment for Growth Before Propagation

1.Area for Growth

You can develop your herbs in any pot-formed vessels that may assist them until once they reap adulthood or you may put together the land for developing with the useful resource of secluding a selected vicinity and plotting the spacing amongst your herbs with the expertise of the dimensions of the vegetation after they attain adulthood to avoid congestion. The ordinary spacing of the plant life could be 10 inches to 16 inches apart which need to make sure enough air and mild to penetrate extensive regions of the plants.

2.Equipment to Acquire

a.For Indoor Growth

●Water-soluble fertilizer; natural rely is most appropriate.

●Fluorescent develop lighting fixtures that provide complete-spectrum moderate at round forty wattages to be located above the growing plant.

●A watering can for irrigation or you may be modern and create an automatic system that would irrigate your flora for you.

●A pesticide that would assist manage pest infestation.

●A cutting device for harvesting.

●Gardening gloves for protection from thorns and splinters.

●A hand trowel for placing seedlings.

b. For Outdoor Growth

●An irrigation device to supply the vegetation with water. This might be someone on a agenda with a watering can who can walk spherical to water the plants or an automatic system that might supply water on command or from following a agenda.

●A pesticide that can help control pest infestation.

●A rake to eliminate stones and other clogs.

●A spade to cast off weeds or to feature cloth to the soil which includes fertilizer.

●A hand trowel for placing seedlings in the ground or for sowing.

●Gardening gloves for protection from thorns and splinters and specific undesirable debris.

●A wheelbarrow to move gardening fabric round.

Conditions to Maintain While Advancing Towards Maturity

- Soil

The seedlings require garden soil it truly is typically loam soil with severa sized minerals of clay, silt, and sand; proportioned with more silt and clay than the sand; and carries some of herbal count number variety which serves as nutrients and supply it a viable texture.

- Fertilizer

Herbs typically do not require heavy fertilizing as this could make the plant leaves and stems make bigger full-size that can purpose a decrease attention of the chemical compounds which the herb is being grown for consequently it is great to paste to herbal don't forget and extremely good moderate fertilizers by myself as a deliver of vitamins for the vegetation if efficiency is of greater importance than quantity. This makes ordinary garden soil blended with a few herbal fertilizer high-quality for outside cultivation. Organic fertilizer is recommended to be added to the soil in liquid layout

(soluble fertilizer in water) each two weeks, very sparingly at the identical time as growing in pots.

- Light

If it is been determined to broaden the herbs interior, then extend lighting fixtures with complete-spectrum

lighting thrusting each heat and cool lighting which mimic solar radiation ought to be positioned above the flora. The maturing seedlings should be stored underneath the slight for up to around 14 hours which want to imitate daytime exposure. Placing the plant life near a window wherein enough sunlight can seep thru to cowl the plant is also viable, but at least six hours of daylight hours publicity an afternoon is wanted for maximum herbs to go through sufficient photosynthesis to live on. Some herbs might also require tons an awful lot less mild exposure than others, for instance; mint, rosemary, and thyme can thrive under drastically low moderate and so it is wonderful to peer a manner to better reveal the vegetation to daytime with minimal electricity wastage. If it is been decided to expand the herbs out of doors, there need to be no obstruction from sunlight hours in the direction of the plant.

- Irrigation

Watering the plant to 3 times in keeping with week have to be enough. The excellent manner to water interior is to permit the pots to dry out slightly in among waterings. To manipulate this well, vicinity a finger inside the pot and it need to be dry at about inches deep. When that is so, then it is first-rate to start watering all over again. The pot normally begins offevolved to dry from the pinnacle and so there want to nevertheless be moisture underneath the pot with a extremely good watering time desk being accompanied. This is carried out to inspire a healthful root system.

(Tip: Do no longer overwater the soil or the vitamins in it will be washed away greater resultseasily.)

(Tip: Do no longer water too short or the water will run via the soil without it absorbing

sufficient of it.)

- Humidity

Hefty airflow everywhere in the plant need to be maintained because the air will supply the plant with humidity which must help keep moisture content material material material immoderate due to the fact the plant can lose moisture through transpiration whilst the air is dry at better prices. Placing the plant underneath a fan or by using the use of a window while indoors can assist with the proper waft of air throughout the plant.

Regular misting of the plant with water have to help sluggish the fee at which flowers transpire.

- Drainage

Herbs grown in pots have to have holes beneath them which need to permit for the soil to dry out as satisfactory herbs like bay, marjoram, oregano, thyme require to have soil this is left to dry barely most of the watering of the pots. Other herbs like rosemary want to never have soil allowed to dry off without a doubt and so it's miles critical to have records on which drainage device is first-rate for the shape of herb you are attempting to develop as many generally tend to rot in excessively wet soil.

- Temperature

Growing herbs need to be stored at temperatures approximated to 21°C at some point of the day and round thirteen°C at some stage in the night time. Some herbs can stay to inform the story temperatures soaring as low as

five°C whilst others like basil cannot live on under 10°C and so research need to be completed on which temperatures the herb you're going to be developing can tolerate.

- Pest Control

If an insect infestation is suspected, then it is quality, to start with, the least toxic and least costly strategies of fertilizing which consist of defensive the leaves of the herbs with a water-cleaning cleansing cleaning soap answer of little soap attention. A 5/four hundred ratio of soap to water answer is generally encouraged.

The software must be finished each week to a degree wherein the pests are not a hassle. If the leaves appear like tormented by the solution, then reduce the cleansing cleaning soap's cognizance in the water to a higher degree. Washing of the plant's leaves need to be accomplished earlier than any form of human consumption as speedy due to the fact the plant has reached adulthood and can be exploited.

A stronger pesticide must artwork with trickier pests which might be proof in competition to the water-cleaning cleaning soap solution, specifically a pesticide that is said to motive the specific pest you noticed.

Harvesting After Complete Gestation Into Maturity

Harvesting of herbs need to be done whilst the plant life have reached a adulthood in which there is a most attention of the compounds liable for the taste and aroma and one-of-a-type fitness benefits of the herb of interest.

With mature annual herbs, as a wonderful deal as 70% in their foliage can be reduce and the plant can hold growing. With perennial herbs, it's far steady to cast off as a good deal as a third of their foliage and the plant will no matter the truth that be able to live on and boom more foliage.

(Tip: Harvest the herbs earlier than vegetation begin to seem as this may are expecting slowing in leaf growth in

the future. Cutting away from plants can help ameliorate the situation; this ought to sell greater leaf boom.)

(Tip: Use sharp tool to reduce away at the foliage whilst harvesting the plant to keep away from tremendous

harm of the plant's xylem tissue and phloem tissue which can be responsible for transporting food compounds, mineral salts, and water from the soil and leaves to all additives of the plant.)

Storing After Harvesting

After harvesting, it's tremendous to take into account which technique will allow your herbs to stay sparkling for longer. How you advocate to apply the herbs in the first region ought to help pinpoint the manner you'll be intending here as well. There are unique sports for a manner you would love to preserve your flowers or how you plan to use them.

1.Drying

Drying can assist boom the awareness of some herbal chemicals you are looking for from the herbs as water will evaporate, despite the fact that with a few one-of-a-kind chemical materials you is probably trying to find; maximum oils will stay as oils evaporate considerably slowly. Knowing which chemical compounds you're after is critical earlier than intending with this technique of protection. Some strategies together with air drying are better than others in terms of retaining natural chemical amount. There are various strategies of doing this.

a.Air Drying

This is considered the conventional approach of drying herbs. It entails putting an collection of harvested herbs in a free bunch and putting them in a skinny, plastic discipline with holes with sufficient air go with the flow, then setting it out to allow drying inside the solar. This technique may be very time-ingesting as it can absorb to a month or occasionally longer for the herbs to dry out truly.

Another way this could be carried out is by scattering the herbs on trays and placing them under the solar this is best to the former when managing leafy herbs.

b. Drying With Heat

This can contain the usage of something from microwaves to ovens to meals dehydrators.

●Using Microwaves

This method is considered volatile as there's a better hazard of the herb charring so it is crucial to set the microwave to supply lower wattages of power; an approximated 800-watt energy supply is most suitable and time frames can variety counting on moisture content fabric and microwave construct; and so, whilst drying, constantly warmness the herb until it reaches a point in which the herb is crumbly, however don't maintain similarly to avoid charring.

●Using Ovens or Food Dehydrators

This method is a lot greater forgiving than using microwaves as there can be lots much less functionality for charring in ovens and meals dehydrators and the process can be more pretty genuinely managed common. A temperature of round eighty°C maintained for two-5 hours can ensure drying to the factor in which the herbs disintegrate with crushing.

For meals dehydrators, following the proprietor's guide recommendations ought to make certain better opportunities of achievement.

2. Freezing

This is taken into consideration to be the easiest manner of storing a herb after harvesting. There can be a trade in look through the years, however flavor content material might be maintained.

It is likewise possible to puree the herbs with minimum water addition after which freeze the paste, then damage the portions of frozen paste and use them later; at the same time as wished.

Chapter 7: Adaptogens

An adaptogen is a selected type of herb this is used for medicinal purposes. For a herb to qualify as an adaptogen it need to be established to be truly secure, non poisonous and function numerous uses that can beautify the health of people taking it. In addition to this they need to assist especially lessen stress; both mentally and physically. As the decision of this sort of herb shows, for a herb to be categorised as an adaptogen it have to will let you adapt.

As with maximum natural treatments, there was large studies into the homes of every herb and the effect on the human body. However, some of the surveys had been carried out within the Soviet Union, Korea and China in the 1980's. The methods and controls used are hard to verify and do inspire humans to talk about on the hassle. In truth, herbal remedies were debated about for many years and probably is probably for plenty extra. Herbal remedies are herbal in spite of the truth that this does not imply they will be regular for intake; that is why it's miles important to speak to a natural expert earlier than you begin taking a brand new natural treatment. The idea of adaptogens emerge as first introduced as extended within the beyond as 1947; it changed into to highlight the consequences of an arterial dilator, on the start advanced in France.

It is idea that many adaptogenic herbs art work thru manner of encouraging and helping the frame to deliver its very personal response to stress or illness. In many approaches that is a form of remedy for individuals who are presently wholesome although may be confused. Stress can regularly be decreased with the aid of surely searching at the every day situations and problems which reason pressure and the splendid techniques of avoiding those situations. The idea of adaptogens may be related to Chinese treatment and plenty of different conventional medicinal methods. They were used for many years to assist people in coping with anxiety, even though there has although been inadequate research regarding how powerful they are.

Regardless of the volume of research, the herbal and mainstream scientific network agree that the subsequent herbs have adaptogenic residences:

•AshwagandhaThis herb is Indian in beginning and has been used for over 3 thousand years. The root of this herb is used and is called a existence extending or rejuvenating agent. It is thought to offer you life itself! This herb is utilized in a giant form of treatments, which incorporates coughs, rheumatism, fatigue, ulcers, sore eyes, inflammations or maybe gynaecological troubles.

Ashwagandha is usually utilized in India by manner of each males and females; it's miles frequently related to improved libido, every other detail of its existence giving homes. In India this herb is so famous that it's miles applied in nearly each form of natural potion, in truth lots of hundreds of this herb are used each year definitely in India.

•EleutheroChinese herbalists confer with the basis of this plant because the Wucha and it is been part of their conventional medicinal practices for over thousand years. In the western international wucha is regularly called Siberian ginseng, although the plant isn't always strictly talking a member of the ginseng family.

The herb grows in Japan, Russia, Korea and most importantly in China. It is said to boost the frame, enhance energy, sexual function, power, and may even decorate your immune system.

Despite initial research there's little recognized approximately how the herb is so effective at improving the fitness of those who take it, despite the fact that studies accomplished in China and Russia shows that it can growth your tolerance to an entire lot of stress factors, collectively with noise, warmth and advanced levels of exercising. It is particularly famous with people who have energetic jobs. Experts advocate that the each day dose need to be between 500 and 1000 milligrams.

•Holy BasilThis herb is truely a member of the mint circle of relatives and intently associated with the sweet basil that you can use in cooking. However, holy basil has been grown for over three thousand years in India and can now be positioned within the majority of tropical international places. It is also known as Tulsi and is considered to be one of the maximum sacred vegetation on India.

The herb is an anti-oxidant and has showed antibacterial, anti-fungal or even anti-inflammatory developments. In conventional remedy it has been used to address the commonplace bloodless as well as Bronchitis, fevers or maybe ulcers or digestive issues.

As with most of the adaptogenic herbs, research is ongoing however early findings seem to verify the existence placing beforehand energy of this herb.

•MacaThis plant is found in the Andes, it is been utilized by the Peruvian people for decades. In reality, there may be proof that shows this herb has been used for over thousand years in the course of Peru and the encircling regions. It is believed to assist your frame in clearing your mind and making you mentally prepared for whatever, it presents a boost on your energy ranges and your libido. It has even been associated with elevated strength and stamina. The plant is frequently combined and then added to any meals of your choosing.

•SchisandraStrictly speaking that may be a berry and no longer a herb, but, it is best used in the manufacturing of medication and its traits and goodness are incredible for the steerage of natural treatments. As a meals supply it is diagnosed to be candy and bitter, at the equal time as being salty, bitter and in lots of techniques tremendously pungent; it isn't a few aspect you will choose out to consume!

The berry comes from a trekking plant which originates from elements of Russia and the northeast of China and is terrific harvested in July or August. The berry is held in rather high regard by the use of individuals who use the conventional Chinese treatment techniques and has an array of powerful advantages.

Due to its taste being typically regular, if now not disgusting, it's miles usually harvested and then dried inside the solar earlier than being introduced it to an entire lot of drug treatments to beautify your electricity. It is feasible to expand this berry almost anywhere, in spite of the fact that, it appears to do better every time it's miles uncovered to bloodless and frosty winters. An alternative to drying it, is to deep refrigerate it and make it proper right into a fitness juice; that is a popular preference of drink in Korea.

The berry has been the mission of many clinical and scientific studies packages and research. There are many warning signs and symptoms and signs that it is incredible at imparting anti inflammatory and antioxidant tendencies that would help to make sure your cells stay healthy and your body glaringly complete of electricity. The ancient Chinese remedy professionals used it to sluggish the growing older system and expand the lifestyles of people who take it. It is also called a sexual tonic and allows to stimulate and increase your natural sexual power.

As well as an first-rate variety of fitness benefits, Schisandra has been researched and has been shown to enhance ranges of interest, patience or even coordination. In impact it'll allow you to supply accurate and immoderate superb work whilst lowering the symptoms and symptoms and symptoms and consequences of highbrow fatigue.

Finally this berry has been used within the development of the anti-hepatitis drug; even in reality taking the berry every day is perception to assist guard your liver from damage. The berry stays distinctly wonderful it many western worldwide places, even though as quickly as people revel in the powerful influences it is probably to turning into an incredibly well-known a part of any fitness regime. To get the endorsed every day dose you without a doubt need to devour maximum of the dried berries; instead you may take the berry indoors a complement to keep away from the particular flavour!

•Rhodiola RoseaThis supplement is also regarded with the aid of using the usage of the names Rhodiola, golden root and rose root. It is grown inside the Siberian and Tian Shan mountains which is probably within the northwest of China. It is a small green plant, but the piece that it beneficial for health and adaptogenic homes is its roots.

It is assumed to offer regular safety toward terrible health, helping the body's herbal defence structures and improving good sized fitness and nicely being. The root has been acknowledged for its capacity to reduce strain and fight fatigue further to to increase strength stages, staying power and stamina. It has moreover historically been used to growth your libido and sexual prowess.

The plant has come below scrutiny with the beneficial useful resource of many scientists because of the truth the compounds which may be determined in it are particular to this shape of plant. The maximum essential compound on this plant is the rosavins; those are a collection of compounds which have been studied and had been associated with the good buy of strain in those who eat them regularly. In fact, the Rhodiola is understood because the brilliant anti-stress complement to be had.

On pinnacle of this, research has verified that Rhodiola can lessen and even get rid of the pressure of having antique with the aid of inhibiting the technique of cellular deterioration. It has moreover been connected with the capacity to improve the endocrine, reproductive and even cardiovascular structures. In truth, whilst monitoring those who have taken this supplement regularly, it is been cited that it is able to assist to enhance their highbrow fitness or maybe their emotional fitness.

As with the diverse dietary dietary supplements that originate from this a part of the area there was a number research performed and the findings are surprising. As nicely as having the capacity to decorate bodily and highbrow fitness it is also a effective sexual aid. Surveys completed inner Russian medical trials confirmed that the herb can enhance the sexual libido; in particular it may help women to emerge as pregnant and clear up many times of erectile sickness. It has even been related with elevated brain function and might counteract the consequences of getting old within the thoughts. Most human beings use this herb in powdered shape, the idea is beaten to achieve this, as little as among 100 fifty and 20 milligrams an afternoon need to be sizeable to look and experience top notch effects.

Choosing an Adaptogen

Your choice may be restricted through your modern fitness or an modern-day medical state of affairs. In the ones times it is crucial to talk to a herbal professional first before trying to find the advice of a systematic expert. They is probably able to direct you towards the outstanding treatment alternatives in your circumstance and the herbal treatments which might be probably to be useful to you. If you are not aware about any gift situations and you are not presently on any treatment then you will be in a feature to speak to a herbal professional who can endorse you which of them ones herbs you need to have. Alternatively you can select one or from this guide and begin taking them at the same time as tracking the changes inside the manner you revel in, behave or maybe react.

An adaptogen is not much like a normal natural remedy; it has the energy to help your frame adapt and enhance its personal capability to deal with the stresses and strains of normal lifestyles. There is an growing amount of research being completed into the recuperation strength of those herbs, this must improve the respectability of this type of treatment and could will let you select the proper natural treatment for your current state of health.

The idea that a natural substance can assist your frame to surely repair its very very very own equilibrium has continuously been a part of the traditional clinical practices inside the Eastern global. The west is now seeing the blessings of this form of remedy and is now discovering and developing its non-public research and studies applications to confirm the recuperation houses of these virtually taking place wonders. As research continues there might be an prolonged information of the complexity of those roots and herbs and the way they're able to beautify your electricity, energy and even your sexual prowess. There are many those who take into account which you do no longer need contemporary-day medicinal drugs a good way to appearance and revel in your high-quality, but, the most practical technique may be to balance your adaptogen consumption alongside side your regular way of life by means of manner of including nutritional dietary dietary supplements in slowly; this can make sure you admire the high-quality effects of each herb.

Chapter 8: Adrenal Glands

The adrenal glands are positioned to your abdomen actually above your kidneys. They are small however are a totally crucial a part of your body. They have severa features but one of the most crucial is the producing of adrenaline, aldosterone and cortisol. These three chemical materials are released in differing amounts in step with what occasions are taking location outside and inside your frame. Cortisol is known as the stress hormone; in instances of stress, it's far launched into your frame and could increase your coronary coronary heart fee, helping to put together your frame for any demanding state of affairs. This natural response allows the 'fight or flight' intuition which every human has. Your reaction can be primarily based totally totally on the hassle you are confronted with and your personal level of confidence on your capabilities to cope with any given scenario. The release of those chemical compounds with the aid of manner of the adrenal glands simply permits your frame to be prepared to react within the way you want.

Unfortunately, current dwelling is extremely disturbing, there are steady problems and motives for your frame to launch those hormones and this could motive a saturation of hormones on your body as well as affecting the capability of the adrenal glands to do their venture well.

The adrenal glands are crafted from additives, the internal, Medulla, is approximately twenty percent of the gland but it's miles as vital as the larger outer layer, the Cortex.

The Medulla

This is the a part of the adrenal gland which regulates your response to stress. These a part of the gland secretes three first-rate chemical substances; which include adrenaline. These chemical compounds are referred to as catecholamines. Whenever the mind perceives a hazard or chance it will robotically deliver a signal to the adrenal glands; the message is straightforward, 'prepare for danger!' The 3 chemical materials are released proper away, they may right away sluggish non-crucial capabilities together with digestion on the identical time as growing blood flow to the mind, muscle mass and make certain you're extra aware about your immediately surroundings. You are then prepared to combat or flee, depending upon the state of affairs. Of course, in modern existence, strain can be because of many incidents so that it will no longer necessitate a physical fight or flee response, which includes giving a public speech or presentation to the board for the number one time. However, the reaction is automated; it is something that used to be an important approach of survival.

The Cortex

This has numerous capabilities, all of which can be in addition as critical due to the truth the function of the medulla:

•Sex Hormones and DHEA are produced by means of the usage of the inner most layer of the cortex. These hormones are critical to the proper functioning of your body. In fact, the male hormone is produced by means of the use of the cortex and can be transformed to testosterone in the testes; even though the male body can produce testosterone immediately from the testes. However, a girl cannot produce the male hormone from every different part of their frame and this makes the adrenal gland specifically important.

•Cortisol is a essential hormone this is produced thru the center section of the cortex. This hormone permits to regulate your sleeping and waking cycle in addition to regulating blood stress, suppressing infection or even assist the body to generate power from food sources which do no longer encompass carbohydrates. It is important to our survival.

•Mineralalocorticoids are produced with the resource of the outer most layer of the cortex and these make sure we secrete the proper amount of fluid and minerals.

Common Issue

A not unusual problem professional thru many human beings on this irritating, cutting-edge global is that the pressure trigger is constantly going; your mind is constantly telling your adrenal glands to secrete the stress hormones and, sooner or later, your deliver of this hormone can not preserve up with the choice for, your reserves turn out to be depleted. This situation is referred to as adrenal fatigue, it is a slow improvement but one this is frequently now not diagnosed until your obtain degree three:

Stage 1

During this diploma you may experience massive wide awake but burdened, you could possibly come upon as having excessive quantities of electricity and capable of undertaking something. Unfortunately, you can moreover be tormented by an lack of ability to sleep properly as your cortisol tiers are unnaturally immoderate inside the night. Thus degree can result in insulin resistance and stomach weight gain.

Stage 2

When you attain this degree you need to haven't any trouble in attending to sleep, but you are in all likelihood to evoke early inside the morning, doubtlessly round 3am and be no longer able to get decrease once more to sleep. This is a quit result of your cortisol manufacturing turning into abnormal. You will usually enjoy tired within the morning and characteristic a upward thrust in energy at some point of the afternoon; frequently a result if a few detail annoying happening. By the night time your cortisol tiers have dropped and you will have little energy or enthusiasm for a few issue.

Step three

Exhaustion! Whether you have slept for 2 hours or fourteen you can feel exhausted! Your coirtisol production can be very low and you will be no longer capable of summon the electricity or enthusiasm to undertake any venture, in spite of the truth that artwork pressures may additionally furthermore pressure you to plod away as first-rate you can. If you acquire this stage you may have an expanded chance of low DHEA or maybe thyroid stages as a manner to offer you a better risk of having autoimmune sickness, which may be pretty risky.

Adrenal fatigue isn't constantly recognized by using using a clinical health practitioner; it is not honestly a recounted scientific state of affairs irrespective of the fact that complete adrenal failure is and adrenal over manufacturing is likewise recounted. Thus can make it difficult to know you have the condition and, in case you do, to recognise what to do approximately it. One if the most critical topics is to reduce the quantity of stress for your existence, you may additionally need to adopt a normal sleep cycle and ensure you workout regularly (regardless of the reality that most effective a bit on the begin). Perhaps the maximum critical lifestyle trade you can make is to have a look at your contemporary food regimen and adjust it. In truth this may suggest switching from any meals you will be sensitive to and that specialize in lean protein. You need to not reduce carbohydrates out as this will make it worse.

Alongside a food plan, the body can gain and healing time can be expanded thru taking natural remedies. There are several alternatives, depending upon which degree of adrenal failure you're stricken by:

Licorice

This is one of the first herbal treatments to function for your food plan, whether or not or now not laid low with level one or degree 3 adrenal fatigue. The herb is concept to encompass triterpenoid saponins that have the functionality to help your body alter the quantity of coristol and cortisone for your body. This will help prevent you from producing excessive quantity so of this hormone, allowing your adrenal glands to get higher.

If you have got an severe case of adrenal fatigue you may be out on a better dose of licorice. However, while taking in large quantities it's far been diagnosed to have an impact at the kidneys, it is able to even cause cortisol to engage with aldosterone receptors that can growth your blood strain through horrifying the sodium and potassium balance on your body. If you're advised to take a excessive dose of licorice you need to be monitored carefully to make certain you aren't setting your fitness similarly at chance.

The recommended every day dose is among and five grams an afternoon; if you are the usage of products that have extracts of licorice you need to consume among twenty five and 75 milligrams in line with day.

As properly as helping you to recover from adrenal fatigue, licorice can help with iron absorption, decrease ranges of coughing, enhancing the steadiness of female hormones and fat modulation. It is also believed that each day consumption of the licorice root will assist the gut lining to heal and reduce the risk of inflammation.

Ginkgo

This natural supplement is likewise called Ginkgo Biloba and is frequently associated with superior circulation and protecting your neuro machine. A a lot much less well known notable of this herb is that it can have a proper away affect on stress tiers. Studies have shown that cortisol tiers drop even as taking a each day dose of ginkgo.

Although it's far believed that this herb improves circulate by means of way of way of thinning the blood, there is no evidence to suggest that this blood thinning influences the capacity for the blood to clot or the risk of a bleed.

Ginkgo is a totally not unusual and without issue available natural supplement; however which means that you can not be taking the same dose as you be given as true with you studied you're in case you buy your supplement from outstanding shops or companies. It can be received in tablet or liquid form and it is best to ensure the dose is standardised; this guarantees you have come to be the identical dose whenever. The advocated each day amount is between a hundred and twenty and 240 milligrams in line with day.

Ashwagandha

This herb, which have become cited in advance inside the ebook, is idea to be beneficial if you have stress brought on drowsing problems. It acts to calm the frame's receptors and decrease cortisol degrees to can help you sleep properly.

More modern-day studies has also determined that this natural complement can beautify the stages of DHEA and testosterone;

this allows to repair depleted levels of those hormones and revitalize your frame.

It may be taken as each a pill or a liquid and it's miles endorsed that, in case you are having dozing problems, you take a few absolutely earlier than bed time. The everyday dose of this is grams according to day of root extract; regardless of the truth that natural experts can recommend as masses as seven grams.

Korean Ginseng

This herbal treatment is likewise called Panax Ginseng and extract of the principle root has been utilized in western treatment practices for decades to address exhaustion; each physical and highbrow. It is likewise a useful herb while dealing with immoderate degrees of stress and troubles together with your immune gadget; every signs of adrenal fatigue. The Chinese have used it for masses of years to restore power and beneficial aid in prolonged residing.

More modern-day studies has demonstrated that it could enhancing insulin sensitivity, enhancing go with the flow or perhaps providing higher reminiscence bear in mind capabilities. It has moreover been associated with repairing broken cells, relieving despair, complications or maybe fatigue. Experts advocate a dose of among one hundred and four hundred milligrams each day, ideally this must be taken in three or 4 doses within the direction of the day to alter the deliver.

Eleuthero

This herb has been proven to assist reduce strain stages via mimicking the stress hormones and growing the extent of safety the frame has from pressure on the equal time as the adrenals have time to refill their assets.

In many strategies this herb is much like Panax Ginseng, however, it is a higher desire for each person who's compelled, especially if they're laid low with recurrent infections and inflammations. It additionally can be used by human beings over forty to help with healthy growing old.

Rhodiola

Recent human trials have hooked up this as an incredibly appropriate herb for reducing moderate despair, stress or maybe fatigue. It is likewise correct at enhancing your mental abilities. A real manner of taking this is to mix it with Ginseng, developing an electricity increase to go along with the good deal of adrenal fatigue symptoms. The encouraged each day quantity is amongst 3 and twelve grams of root extract.

Rehmannia

This herb has very comparable homes to licorice. It is thought to useful aid anyone suffering with depletion of the adrenal glands or fatigue, similarly to immune gadget problems. Daily intake want to be about four grams to provide the most ideal effects.

Astragalus

This herb is often used alongside facet Rehmannia and Eleuthero as it works as each a tonic for advanced fitness and as a guide for the adrenal glands; supporting them to recover from overuse.

The herb can assist to modify boom hormone ranges, blood glucose degrees, blood waft or even blood strain. It furthermore assists with water balance and the cut price of inflammations. Experts advise taking among 2.Five and three.Four grams constant with day and the affects ought to be awesome inner a few weeks.

It is critical to take a look at that each one the herbs listed can be taken independently of every tremendous or they may be combined to offer the excellent feasible chance of a short healing from adrenal fatigue. Before you begin to combination the herbs it's miles truly beneficial to gain professional recommendation. If this is not an preference the following tips may additionally additionally additionally help:

•Licorce is the quickest running herb and will offer without delay treatment further to essential improvements to your fitness.

•Ginkgo will beautify your skip and the amount of oxygen getting round your body. It additionally gives brilliant anti-oxidant safety.

•Ashwagandha will restore your internal center. You will see brief improvements on your strength, libido and stamina.

•Korean Ginseng is notion to guide every adrenal and thyroid capabilities in the body.

•Ashwagandha and Ginseng make an cheap mixture that lets in you to revitalise you and assist your adrenals to get higher.

Chapter 9: The Thyroid Gland

This gland can be placed at the base of your neck, it's miles butterfly shaped and it's miles liable for controlling the deliver if hormones in your body which modify your metabolism. Generally the quicker your metabolism the better succesful you may be to convert food into energy. An loss of functionality to adjust your metabolism properly have to bring about a sluggish metabolism so that it will depart you feeling tired and lacking in electricity.

The thyroid is an essential part of your body, the hormones it produces help to modify most of the maximum crucial abilties of your frame, at the side of:

•Breathing

•Heart rate

•Muscle power

•Body weight

•Menstrual cycles

•Cholesterol tiers

•Body temperature

•The frightened device.

The thyroid lies on every element of your windpipe, linked with the resource of using a strip of tissues called the isthmus. It is possible for the 2 halves not to be associated; the function of the thyroid may be unimpaired. The number one hormones made via the thyroid gland are:

•Triiodothyroninethat is referred to as the lively hormone and makes up twenty percentage of the thyroid production.

•Thyroxinethis makes up the opportunity eighty percentage.

The quantity of these two hormones released and the timing in their release is managed through the hypothalamus gland and the pituitary gland. These glands are in the mind and talk with every distinctive; the hypothalamus tells the pituitary whether or not or now not to launch greater or lots much less of the 2 hormones listed above. This guarantees the frame's supply of those hormones remains even at a few degree in the day, no matter what interest you are undertaking.

Unfortunately there are numerous motives why the thyroid may also furthermore no longer produce enough, or it may even produce too much of one or both hormones. There are severa symptoms that allows you to provide a clue that the difficulty lies with the thyroid gland:

If you have got had been given an excessive amount of of those hormones to your body you're likely to reveal the subsequent signs and symptoms and signs and symptoms:

•Anxious, irritable or definitely moody.

•Hyperactive

•Nervous, which includes having shaking hands.

•Sweating or turning into particularly touchy to immoderate temperatures.

•Loss of hair

At the opposite give up of the size you may now not be generating sufficient of those hormones, if this is the case you may have a few or all of the following symptoms and signs:

•Tiredness notwithstanding the fact which you also are probable to have hassle dozing as your frame struggles to regulate itself.

•You will discover it difficult to pay attention on anything for additonal than a couple of minutes.

•You may enjoy depressed.

•Your hair and pores and pores and skin will appear dry; even in case you use day by day moisturiser.

•Your joints and even your muscle companies end up painful.

•You becomes touchy to cold temperatures.

Testing

Your clinical doctor may be able to run a series of checks which could determine whether or not or not you've got an issue together with your thyroid gland. The tests might also moreover even display whether or not the gland is diseased or if the pituitary gland isn't jogging well. If the pituitary gland is not operating nicely it is probably that there may be one-of-a-kind issues because it influences extraordinary components of your body. There are many reasons why the thyroid gland is not going for walks properly and your medical doctor might be able to perform numerous exams to affirm the problem.

The maximum common reasons of thyroid issues are:

•Toxicityspecially a few kind of publicity which has broken the gland, which incorporates radiation or heavy metal.

•DeficiencyLow levels of iodine and / or selenium may have an impact on the potential of the thyroid gland to provide hormones.

•Food Sensitivity and intolerancegluten and A1 casein allergies will prevent your body from producing sufficient ranges of hormones.

•Hormone Imbalance —this is covered in greater detail inside the subsequent bankruptcy however a hormone imbalance will save you the mind from issuing the proper instructions to the glands and motive a thyroid problem.

Herbal treatments

Doctors will prescribe masses of prescription medicinal drugs to help the thyroid paintings well or to update the position of the thyroid. They may check out in addition to select out and, with a piece of good fortune resolve, any underlying trouble. However, there are numerous natural treatments that might assist to stability your body and make sure your thyroid is jogging properly:

Rehmannia

This herb has been tested to have a effective impact at reducing infection inside the frame. A thyroid gland which is not jogging well is probable to be infected and this herb will assist to relieve this symptom. It is also packed entire of vitamins A, B, C and D and has been used historically with great achievement for assisting balance your hormones.

Schisandra

This plant and its berries had been proven to guard your frame from antioxidants. Research has additionally established that this herb can help to enhance the functioning of your stressful device, immune device, respiration device and your cardiovascular device. It may additionally moreover even help to save you excessive blood sugar tiers. It is not diagnosed precisely how this herb works but it is hoped that greater research will help to enlighten natural and clinical practitioners.

Rhodiola

This herb is understood to growth your fats burning capability and enhance your thoughts electricity. It can even increase your power levels! It has been counseled that this herb is robust at reducing the opportunities of contracting most cancers, stopping melancholy and improving each the cardiovascular machine and the primary worried device. It is also relatively appropriate at protecting the strain reaction structures on your frame, allowing them time to recover at the same time as permitting you and your body to get over the underlying reason. The perception is that, using a herb like this one, together with a balanced weight-reduction plan and exercise, you will be capable of relieve the pressure to your body and it will natural pass decrease back to a balanced country; even the thyroid gland can start to artwork typically once more.

Bacopa

Research has tested that this herb has a proper away affect at the thyroid gland, growing the manufacturing of Tyroxine without affecting the alternative chemical compounds and hormones within the body. In effect, this herb will without delay stimulate your thyroid gland and may be an amazing accomplice in the fight in competition to an underactive thyroid.

Bladderwrack

This herb is in truth a seaweed with adaptogenic homes. It is idea by way of manner of severa particular names, consisting of rockweed, sea very wellor even bladder fucus. It become first placed in 1811 and is a natural deliver of iodine. If your thyroid trouble stems from a deficiency of iodine then this is the correct answer as it will boom your iodine tiers evidently. In fact, many human beings have used this herb to grade by grade prevent taking synthetic thyroid dietary supplements. If centered on Ashwaganda it has really been recognized to stimulate the manufacturing of thyroid in the frame. It is important to examine that bladderwrack harvested from the open sea will were open to feasible contaminants, which consist of heavy metals that could make a thyroid problem worse. It is, consequently, important to gain the seaweed from an accepted provider.

Black Walnut

This species of tree is a part of the walnut own family and flowers often. It has been known as a most cancers treatment as research has demonstrated it's far able to killing a parasite this is notion to reason a few cancers. The nuts are wealthy in omega three and nutrition C and are seemed to improve the health of the gut lining. It is likewise a wealthy supply of iodine.

Echinacea

Whilst this herb is thought for its anti-inflammatory competencies, it's also outstanding at anti-viral and ache alleviation.

The herb may be harvested at almost any time but the time and part of the plant getting used will manage the impact that it has. Early plants may be harvested and could help the function of a wholesome immune system. Meanwhile roots which might be harvested in the autumn will provide a healthy inflammatory device, the ones are particularly effective at the same time as dealing with sinus issues and need to be used at the start of an hassle; no longer s a long time solution. It has been confirmed to have a super effect on thyroid deficiencies and isn't always going to purpose any autoimmune troubles.

Eleuthero

This herb has been used for hundreds of years in Chinese medicinal drug to reduce the effects of strain with the useful resource of way of growing the capability of the frame to deal with those issues. Whilst this herb does no longer have an instantaneous have an impact on at the thyroid gland it's miles terrific at balancing the relaxation of the frame and decreasing the strain the body is under; allowing the thyroid to begin strolling properly once more.

Coleus For Skohlii

This has historically been used to deal with coronary heart disorder, convulsions, peculiar and ordinary ache and, even, troubles with urination. It is a effective herb which has been acknowledged to encourage and enhance cellular fitness; this improves the messages which is probably carried throughout the frame and ensure all frame cells are able to burn their stored fats.

Hawthorn Leaf and Berry

This herb has been verified to be powerful at treating congestive coronary coronary coronary heart failure, angina or perhaps immoderate blood stress. It is thought that a healthful coronary coronary heart leads to a healthy endocrine system which guarantees the frame s balanced and hormones are produced at the right degrees. This stability will make sure that the thyroid has enough hormones to complete its activity properly. It is likewise rich in antioxidants; the particles for your frame which discover and damage loose radicals. This is crucial as free radicals can purpose mobile demise or even tamper together with your DNA.

Lemon Balm

This herb is a part of the mint family and is idea to have a calming impact on the frame; thoughts and soul. It is also seemed to act at once at the thyroid gland and it has been suggested that it could block some of the hobby of the thyroid hormone. Reducing this interest and manufacturing makes it a very a fulfillment herb at the same time as dealing with an overactive thyroid gland.

Bugleweed

This is an preference for individuals who do now not want to take prescription anti-thyroid capsules. It is unsure if the natural acids in this herb artwork to block the gland from receiving commands to provide hormones or of it absolutely works with the useful resource of manner of preventing the entrance of these hormone triggers into the thyroid gland.

You most effective want to eat a small amount of this herb each day to advantage the first-rate results. It seems to have an impact at the ability of the body to soak up iodine making it tougher to make immoderate quantities of the thyroid hormone.

Commiphora Mukul

The resinous sap from this plant is known as gum guggul and the extract from this gum is used to convert thyroxine into Triiodothyronine. This lets in it to decorate the quantity of thyroid manufacturing with out regarding the pituitary gland and complicate the body. This herb is mainly effective as many thyroid issues are related to the thyroid gland and not the pituitary gland.

Experts propose one hundred milligrams in step with day.

Notes

It is essential to take a look at which you need to recognise whether or not or now not your thyroid gland is generating an excessive amount of or too little hormones. Both problems are treatable however they want to be addressed in another way. Underactive thyroids may be stimulated thru prescription drugs or you may even administer a artificial drug to update it. Overactive thyroids want to be depressed, the production should be decreased. This is typically more hard to reap than 'topping up' your hormone production. Herbal remedies might also motive the thyroid to prevent manufacturing be desensitising the receptors. Alternatively they'll paintings to convey the complete body lower back into stability and treatment the middle difficulty. Herbal drug treatments have their origins in ancient China; in this lifestyle it changed into believed that every residing element wishes stability; the Yin and the Yang. This approach to medication is instrumental to the administration of herbal remedies; current research shows how a achievement some of those herbs can be at rebalancing the body. As constantly, are seeking out recommendation from a scientific doctor and a natural expert before blending herbs and prescription medicinal drugs.

Chapter 10: Balancing your Hormones

Balanced hormones are vital to being able to cope with all of the exquisite factors of a 'regular' existence. There are consistent pressures from all instructions which want to be dealt with, this may make it very hard to live on pinnacle of everything and bear in mind in yourself. In truth, all people's hormones change as they age. It is customary that kids getting into formative years may have raging hormones as they discover greater concerning the area around them. It is likewise an normal, despite the truth that frequently misunderstood, part of a women's life that they may undergo hormonal changes in their forties or fifties.

Many people see hormonal modifications in a horrific mild, however they may be definitely an vital part of maturing and growing older. Your hormones are your body's manner of handling an entire lot of situations; some of that might pretty worrying. The sensitive balance of hormone manufacturing can be knocked out of sync through catching a common cold, or some distinctive slight infection. You may not expect some thing of it and the outcomes may be small, but the truth of the trouble is that our our our our bodies are dramatically suffering from all the activities and pollutants spherical us every day.

Small modifications, at the side of those above, will generally kind themselves out after the contamination or brief event has passed. However, every so often the hormonal trade does now not balance itself. If you have got were given the following signs and symptoms, you probable have a hormone hassle:

•Weight Gain

There are many reasons you may advantage weight, however, if you find that there is a persistent weight gain and that you are exercise often and consuming properly, you may be suffering from a hormone imbalance. Small adjustments for your food plan can help.

•Belly fat

Alongside weight gain you could moreover find out that you are collecting weight around your belly. This is generally a reaction with the aid of using your body to pressure; it will overproduce a few hormones and beneath produce others. Your frame will react to the ones changes by way of way of using storing fats to your belly; in case it's far wanted.

•Decreased Libido

Hormonal imbalance generally consequences in an loss of capacity to sleep nicely. In flip this will have an effect to your potential to provide the intercourse hormone and your desire for intercourse and reduce or possibly vanish!

•Tiredness

Tiredness can be a signal of a awful diet; an excessive amount of sugar will result in peaks and troughs in some unspecified time in the future of the day. However, it can moreover be the quit result of hormonal adjustments. If simple dietary changes do not have an effect in your capability to live awake then you'll be tormented by a hormonal imbalance so that you can want correcting.

•Irritable

If you genuinely experience out of kinds, likely disturbing, depressed or perhaps stressed all of the time you're possibly to be suffering from a hormonal imbalance. It is pretty likely that your body is overworked and not receiving the critical nutrients and minerals which can be critical to a healthy frame and mind. It is vital to take a breather out of your traumatic life every now and then and stability your hormones.

•Insomnia

Not napping for prolonged enough or having notably disrupted sleep cycles will start to have an impact on your cortisol tiers. This has a proper away have an effect on on your hormone levels in addition to affecting many different components of your fitness. If you are struggling to sleep properly or in any respect you can ensure your hormone degrees are unbalanced.

•Sweating

Sweating at night time time time and hot flushes are usually associated with women going thru the menopause. They are in fact signs and symptoms of the hormonal modifications which might be going on in their our bodies at the moment. If you begin to enjoy these signs and signs and symptoms and signs, whether or not going via the menopause or no longer, you already know your frame is hormonally imbalanced.

Instead of starting on hormone opportunity treatment it's miles a incredible concept to have a examine the food you devour and to establish which natural treatments will benefit you the most. Emotional issues can also purpose the latest flushes and sweating and it's miles nicely surely really worth thinking about what feelings have been going through your head as your temperature rose.

•Digestive troubles

If you phrase which can be becoming bloated often or that your digestive tool is slowing down you could well assume which you are rushing your food or not chewing it up well. However, this will virtually be an problem with a hormonal imbalance. Insufficient hormones on your body can save you your digestive device from being capable of take within the nutrients you want. In effect your body is starving irrespective of what you devour.

•Cravings

You can also additionally furthermore maintain to consume a few factor extended whilst you're entire after which pause and ask your self why. The answer is not absolutely which you loved it! Overeating is a form of craving which may be linked to adrenal fatigue and insulin resistance; it's far simply a hormone imbalance that's inflicting it! The first step in correcting this imbalance is to reduce your sugar intake. You will then be capable of have a observe what herbal treatments can help in resolving your underlying hassle.

There are many unique options of herbs and combos which may be added to your diet to help your body balance its hormone tiers. You may additionally additionally need to undertake an ordeal and mistakes method to discover the right aggregate that works brilliant for you, the advice of a herbalist can also be beneficial.

The following herbs are generally very effective at assisting you to stability your hormone degrees:

Maca Root

This herb is also called Lepidium meyenii and is understood to have a pleasant effect on your hormone ranges. It has moreover been proven to be beneficially when dealing with infertility, low strength ranges, ordinary moods and it will even help your libido! One have a have a look at has even tested that during case you eat healthy for human consumption maca, (maca which has been cooked and dried), it can have a very powerful impact on menopausal girls. It has been verified to reduce warm flushes, night time time sweats or maybe tension, melancholy and coronary heart palpitations. It is usually encouraged that you start with a small dose of this effective herb, the herb will relieve the stress your frame is presently under thru relieving the signs of pressure on your body and allowing your adrenal glands to get better.

Maca does now not proper away have an effect on the hormones in your frame; however it does offer pretty a range of vitamins, which encompass calcium, phosphorous, weight-reduction plan B1 and food plan B12. These nutrients are utilized by the endocrine which ultimately permits to stability the hormones for your frame.

Chasteberry

This is the fruit of the chaste tree and is also referred to as Vitex and Agnus Castus. The chaste tree is generally positioned in most vital Asia and plenty of factors of the Mediterranean. Research shows that this berry has been used for hundreds of years thru girls; it is stated to relieve menstrual troubles and assist women produce breast milk. It can also reduce breast ache, edema, constipation or maybe complications.

The fruit if this tree is believed to have an effect at the pituitary gland and may help to modify the frame's metabolism, the immune gadget or even encourage right improvement of the pancreas.

Black Cohosh

This herb has been used for over hundred years and is idea to help deal with menopausal symptoms. It has furthermore been used successfully to reduce inflammation, especially on the same time because it's been due to osteoarthritis, rheumatoid arthritis and neuralgia. It has moreover been associated with having estrogenic traits and it is believed that the mixture of these capabilities work in the body to assist regulate your hormones and convey the frame all over again into stability.

Saw Palmetto

This herb has been used to successfully deal with noncancerous boom of the prostate gland. This is one if the herbs it's researched and examined on men similarly to women. Many of the herbs which cope with hormone imbalance are targeted at girls as they're state of affairs to huge modifications of their hormones when they input the menopause. However, guys can also be afflicted with the aid of hormonal imbalance and this herb has proved to be in particular particular at balancing hormone levels. A side effect of using this herb to treat an enlarged prostate is a stated improvement in the urinary tract and the go with the flow from this tract.

The herb has moreover been related with a discount in instances of male pattern baldness. It is frequently combined with nettle extract and has validated to advantage fulfillment in improving the hormonal stability in males and females.

Asian Ginseng

The root of this herb is applied in a big variety of diverse natural treatments. It will check the hormonal stability of your body and act at the strain receptors to assist correct them. It does act via using the use of growing pressure type issues in the body however these will now not be affecting your hormonal balance. It can be taken in a whole lot of precise methods, which encompass any form of drink or as a pill.

Ashwagandha

This herb is noted frequently during the ebook as it's miles applicable to the treatment of a good sized type of various conditions. It is, in effect, a terrific herb although it has a very bitter flavor; it's miles advocated to eat it as part of every a drink or a few meals. Taking it via a pill is also an super alternative. This herb has been utilized by opportunity medical practitioners and the more traditional medical medical doctors for decades; it is relied on to assist in masses of instances and has been mounted to help balance hormones via alleviating the strain for your frame.

Dong Quai

This herb originates from Japan, China and Korea. It is technically a part of the parsley family and has a bittersweet flavor. This makes it pretty smooth to consume. Research and studies have verified it to be an powerful way of balancing your hormones; whether or not male or woman.

Chapter 11: Popular Herbal treatments and Treatments

The first rate time to begin taking a natural complement is earlier than you're suffering with hormonal imbalance, adrenal fatigue or every extraordinary form of conditions which can be treated via the usage of herbal medication. Unfortunately most human beings do not recall the preventative help which herbs can offer them with until they really need the herbs to get better. Despite an boom within the sort of clinical specialists who're organized to preserve in mind opportunity drug remedies, the same old method to fitness care stays a visit to your scientific health practitioner, determined by a prescription and likely study up visits and brilliant drug remedies. Only while the identical antique method isn't always running do humans take into account what options are to be had.

Herbs can offer a possible possibility to prescription drugs, often preventing you from wanting a lifetime of dependence on the ones drugs. They can also assist to prevent quite some illnesses and assist in crucial a complete and healthful life.

The following herbal treatments are the maximum common and well-known ones for managing pretty some illnesses and problems:

Turmeric

This spice is often utilized in curries although you may upload it to almost any dish you need to. The spice includes a substance known as curcumin it truly is thought to be an super anti-inflammatory. It is fairly effective at lowering the swelling and irritation which due to arthritis.

The cutting-edge day research moreover indicates that curcumin can lessen the size of precancerous legions called colon polyps. If this substance is taken alongside facet a pinch of quercetin, the studies showed that the average variety of polyps reduced via using an high-quality sixty percentage on the equal time as people who remained shrank to as a minimum 1/2 of in their real duration.

It has additionally been linked with decreasing the opportunity of Alzheimer's because it clears the plaques which shape on the mind and are a longtime feature of the scenario. Experts propose 400mg of curcumin and 20mg of quercetin taken 3 instances an afternoon for max have an effect on.

Cinnamon

Research shows that folks who consume simply 1g of cinnamon a day will lessen their blood sugar level with the useful resource of manner of ten percentage, lowering the threat or the effects of type 2 diabetes.

Cinnamon is also effective at reducing ldl ldl cholesterol, a dose of 6mg constant with day has been established to reduce the quantity of amount of ldl ldl cholesterol inside the frame thru as plenty as 13 percentage. It additionally reduced the quantity of triglycerides via way of a large twenty three percentage. Both of those substances boom within the body and boom your threat of coronary coronary heart sickness or stroke.

Cinnamon is an remarkable desire to reduce the possibility of this taking place; but, it is critical to word that an excessive amount of of the spice in its natural united states is terrible in your fitness. You have to take cinnamon in a liquid shape to maximize the blessings and avoid any dangers.

Rosemary

This herb is often used as a garnish in a dish; usually it's miles sincerely to make the meal appearance applicable. However it can additionally provide a number of health advantages. Frying, broiling or even grilling meat will create heterocyclic amines; those are known as cancer agents and had been related to severa cancers. However, if you add rosemary extract on your meat earlier than cooking it's going to appreciably reduce the amount of cancer causing agents because it destroys them at some stage in the cooking gadget.

Rosemary it is fed on has moreover been related with a decrease inside the type of carcinogens bonding with the DNA on your body. Research has validated that this bonding is step one in tumour formation, preventing this from occurring is a first-rate leap ahead for scientific research despite the fact that the research ought to be continued to affirm the consequences.

The awesome manner to feature rosemary to your food regimen is to marinate your meat earlier than cooking. This may be in any kind of sauce as prolonged because it has rosemary in it.

Ginger

This normal looking plant has been related with preventing nausea for many years. People who be afflicted by sea sickness will frequently be advised to try eating ginger biscuits or cake in advance than they excursion. In reality ginger does extra than assist with nausea, it is been proven to be extraordinary at calming a massive range of belly upsets, even those due to being pregnant or chemotherapy.

Ginger acts via the use of blocking off the results of a chemical called serotonin that is produced via the utilization of each the stomach and the thoughts at the same time as you are feeling nauseous; it additionally stops the production of loose radicals, effectively putting off the upset stomach earlier than it even starts offevolved.

Studies have confirmed 500mg of ginger, taken every four hours is as effective as any over-the-counter medicinal drug. You can opt to take more, even doubling the dose of ginger and the consequences might be appreciably better than an over the counter medicine.

Consuming ginger has moreover been related with a lower in blood strain, arthritis pain or perhaps the chance of most cancers. This is due to the fact it is an anti-inflammatory and this allows to lessen the ache due to swollen joints in arthritis sufferers. It lets in the body to alter blood float that is in all likelihood to decrease your blood strain.

The modern-day-day studies even indicates that powdered ginger is more powerful than chemotherapy at killing ovarian maximum cancers cells. This may be actual for specific kinds of cancers as well, regardless of the reality that further trying out is wanted as all research up to now has been finished in test tubes internal a laboratory.

Holy Basil

Basil is a not unusual cooking factor; however its cousin, Holy Basil is much less broadly diagnosed however may additionally furthermore have exceptional fitness advantages to offer.

Holy Basil works to your body via developing the stages of adrenaline and noradrenaline at the same time as reducing the serotonin degrees. This combination will lessen your feelings of pressure and assist to calm your body; much less pressure equates to a massive form of health benefits internal your body. Holy Basil works to get rid of headaches and indigestion as well.

Studies have already been done in mice which decided that a tea made from holy basil have turn out to be effective at shrinking tumours and decreased the blood supply to those tumours stopping their spread. The tumours it's been examined on thus far are those which purpose breast maximum cancers. There is lots more trying out and studies to do but a massive amount of capability with this herb.

You will likely need to big order the herb as it is not commonly at your neighborhood plant shop. The excellent manner to eat it's miles with the resource of manner of brewing about ten leaves in cups of boiling water for 5 mins.

St. John's Wort

This herb has been used for decades to save you depression and relieve tension. It has been shown to be as effective as the majority of drugs available to be had available on the market and does no longer have any of the element outcomes related to prescribed drugs.

It is likewise feasible that it will permit you to to sleep better. The herb includes a substance known as melatonin. This substance already takes location for your frame and allows to alter your sleep cycle. Taking St. John's Wort will growth the amount for your bloodstream and persuade your frame to make extra! The quit end result can be a better night time time's sleep.

It is commonly endorsed that you take 300mg 3 times a day to make certain you got the maximum benefit from this powerful herb. However, it's been placed to have an effect on a few prescription drug remedies and also you ought to test collectively with your physician earlier than beginning to take it.

Garlic

Garlic changed into traditionally used to maintain off vampires! However, it additionally has been proven to correctly decrease the threat of maximum cancers. In particular the studies has visible a drop in costs of ovarian and colorectal cancers.

A clinical trial finished in Japan noticed a dramatic good buy in the length and big type of colon polyps noticed through clinical docs. The trial subjects were all patients who had a facts of colon polyps.

Garlic additionally contains allicin which has been associated with reduced blood strain; in fact research suggest that this substance, placed in garlic, should drop excessive blood strain through the use of as an awful lot as thirty factors. A separate take a look at confirmed that garlic can be instrumental in slowing arterial blockages that could help to save you strokes.

The excellent way of obtaining the right degree of garlic is with the aid of the usage of taking a 1000mg tablet that is elderly garlic extract. To gain the identical impact with smooth garlic you may need to eat 5 cloves a day!

Green Tea

This herb has been used as part of every Chinese and India medicinal practices for loads of years. The tea comes from the leaves of the shrub Camellia Sinensis which turn out to be in the beginning grown in South East Asia but is now located in places all through the entire global. The leaves and leaf buds are dried to make the tea.

It is whole of antioxidants which destroys the free radicals on your frame. This lets in to reduce the signs and signs and symptoms of getting older and lets in save you harm on your eyes as you age.

More current studies show that a chemical positioned in green tea can certainly block specific molecules from developing into lung maximum cancers. It has even been demonstrated to inhibit or dramatically lessen the speed at which tumour cells develop. It is also an effective anti-bacterial drink and it stimulates the immune machine to make certain it is ready and able to fight off infection. It is even capable of reducing dental plaque. Further research have verified it to be effective at lowering immoderate blood strain and excessive levels of cholesterol as well as helping the body to alter blood sugar tiers.

It is one of the extraordinary herbs that have a massive variety of benefits and no discernable facet effects.